Osteoporosis
A Guide for Health-care Professionals

Osteoporosis

A Guide for Health-care Professionals

ANNE SUTCLIFFE BSc(HONS), RGN, DN, HV
Osteoporosis Specialist Nurse

WHURR PUBLISHERS
LONDON AND PHILADELPHIA

Other Wiley Editorial Offices

John Wiley & Sons Inc., 111 River Street, Hoboken, NJ 07030, USA

Jossey-Bass, 989 Market Street, San Francisco, CA 94103-1741, USA

Wiley-VCH Verlag GmbH, Boschstr. 12, D-69469 Weinheim, Germany

John Wiley & Sons Australia Ltd, 42 McDougall Street, Milton, Queensland 4064, Australia

John Wiley & Sons (Asia) Pte Ltd, 2 Clementi Loop #02-01, Jin Xing Distripark, Singapore 129809

John Wiley & Sons Canada Ltd, 22 Worcester Road, Etobicoke, Ontario, Canada M9W 1L1

Wiley also publishes its books in a variety of electronic formats. Some content that appears in print may not be available in electronic books.

A catalogue record for this book is available from the British Library

ISBN -13   978-0-470-01967-2
ISBN -10   0-470-01967-0

Printed and bound in the UK by TJ International Ltd, Padstow, Cornwall

Contents

Preface

Osteoporosis is a disorder characterized by compromised bone strength that predisposes to an increased risk of fracture. It has been estimated that one in three women and one in twelve men in the UK will experience an osteoporosis-related fracture during their lifetime. These fractures are associated with excess mortality, substantial morbidity, and major health and social expenditure. The incidence of the disease has increased steadily in the latter half of the twentieth century, and will continue to do so in this millennium as the number of elderly people rises.

In the past osteoporosis was regarded as an inevitable consequence of ageing aggravated by the menopause in women. Diagnostic techniques were poor and treatment options were limited. Over the last two decades there has been a great increase in the knowledge and understanding of the scientific and clinical aspects of this condition.

Osteoporosis has been more clearly defined and our understanding of its pathophysiology and epidemiology is now more refined. Significant advances have developed in the prediction of risk and the identification of those most likely to be at risk of fractures. Rapid assessment and multidisciplinary management of the patient who has sustained a fracture are essential to promote favourable outcomes. Prevention involves maximizing bone strength through adequate nutrition and exercise on a lifelong basis. With respect to elderly people, falls prevention will also aid in fracture reduction. There have been technical improvements and advances in methods of measuring bone density, enabling both case finding and the monitoring of response to treatment. Although effective treatment options that reduce bone loss and fracture risk exist, it is clear that there are problems with both under-diagnosis and long-term adherence.

The management of osteoporosis and its related fractures spans diverse areas of health care, including rheumatology, orthopaedics, endocrinology, care of elderly people and primary care. To focus on early assessment, prevention, diagnosis and treatment, it is necessary to engage doctors, nurses and other health-care professionals. Having worked as a specialist nurse in this field for many years, I am aware that the broad spectrum of nursing provides an ideal arena where nurses are well placed to aid in the management of this condition. The aims of this book are to provide an overview of the important aspects of osteoporosis, and facilitate understanding of the concepts and processes involved, thus establishing a sound knowledge base that may be translated into optimum care throughout all nursing disciplines.

Anne Sutcliffe

CHAPTER 1

Pathogenesis of osteoporosis

- Bone is a living, dynamic tissue
- Bone remodelling provides a mechanism for self-repair and adaptation to stress
- Peak bone mass and onset of bone loss are major determinants of future fracture risk
- Attainment of bone mass and onset of bone loss are influenced by many factors

The risk of osteoporosis depends in part upon skeletal development, the attainment of peak bone mass and the amount of bone lost in later life. Disruption of the processes that normally maintain skeletal balance and turnover will lead to incompetence and osteoporosis. This chapter reviews the development and maintenance of skeletal mass and the factors that determine the gain and loss of bone throughout life.

Although the popular image of the skeleton is of an inert, hard structure supporting the rest of the body, bone is a dynamic tissue that undergoes constant remodelling throughout life. It is metabolically active, continually being formed and resorbed by bone cells, the activity of which is modified by many factors. This remodelling is necessary to allow the skeleton to increase in size during growth, respond to the physical stresses placed on it, and repair structural damage caused by fatigue or fracture. In addition to its mechanical properties, bone also plays an important role in calcium homeostasis. It contains 99% of the total body calcium and phosphate, providing a large mineral reservoir that can be drawn upon to maintain normal calcium balance.

Bone composition and structure

The skeleton comprises two types of bone (Figure 1.1): cortical or compact, and trabecular or cancellous bone. Cortical bone, which forms about 80% of the skeleton, is predominantly found in the shafts of the long bones and surfaces of flat bones. It is composed of compact bone laid down around central canals (haversian systems) which contain blood and lymphatic vessels, nerves and connective tissue. Trabecular bone is mainly located in the inner parts of flat bones and at the ends of long bones, where it forms a lattice-like structure within bone. Trabecular bone has a larger surface area and undergoes greater remodelling, and is therefore more responsive to changes in mineral metabolism than cortical bone.

Bone comprises an organic matrix, a mineral phase and bone cells. Most of the matrix is composed of collagen fibres that account for 65% of the total organic component of bone tissue. This fibrous organic matrix gives bone its resistance to tractional and torsional forces. Osteocalcin is predominantly confined to bone and accounts for up to 20% of the non-collagenous proteins. Other non-collagenous proteins found in bone include glycoproteins, the most relevant being alkaline phosphatase, osteonectin and cell attachment proteins. Bone matrix also contains growth factors that play an important regulatory role in bone modelling and remodelling; these include transforming growth factors, platelet-derived growth factors, insulin-like growth factor, endothelial growth factor and bone morphogenetic proteins.

The mineralization of bone leading to compressive strength and rigidity begins with the precipitation of calcium and phosphate ions that begin to induce crystallization. As crystal growth occurs, mineralization spreads, resulting in the formation of mature, fully calcified bone, known as hydroxyapatite. This process is also underpinned by magnesium, small amounts of sodium and traces of fluoride.

Bone cells

Cells with distinct functional features cover all bone surfaces. These include osteoclasts, osteoblasts and osteocytes, with other cell types in the bone microenvironment playing an additional role in the regulation of bone remodelling.

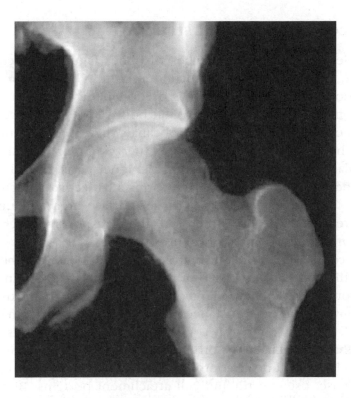

Figure 1.1 Types of bone: cortical – 80% of skeleton, with slow turnover; trabecular – 20% of skeleton, with rapid turnover.

Osteoclasts are efficient multinucleate cells, derived from precursors of the monocyte–macrophage lineage; their lifespan and ultimate fate remain uncertain. The osteoclast degrades bone by attaching to a bone surface and secreting acids and enzymes into the mineralized bone surface (Suda et al. 1992). They are mobile cells and after eroding one pit in mineralized bone they may move to another site. Osteoblasts that descend from bone marrow-derived stem cells are the bone-forming cells. They synthesize collagen and other proteins and have an important role in the subsequent mineralization of the bone matrix (Owen 1985). Osteocytes are mature osteoblasts that become trapped within calcified bone. They play an important role in the osteogenic response to mechanical stimuli, 'sensing' physical strains and initiating an appropriate modelling or remodelling response via the production of a cascade of chemical messengers (Lanyon 1992).

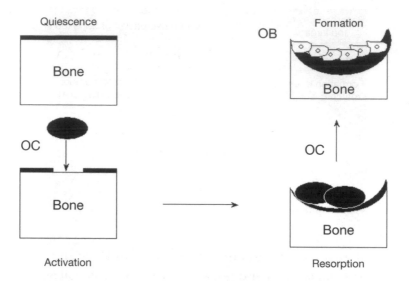

Figure 1.2 Bone remodelling. OB, osteoblast; OC, osteoclast.

Bone remodelling (Figure 1.2)

In the mature adult, skeletal size is neither increasing nor decreasing but bone is continuously being turned over. This process termed 'bone remodelling' provides a mechanism for self-repair and adaptation to stress. Occurring in both cortical and trabecular bone, it takes place at discrete sites on the bone surface, described as bone remodelling units. The process consists of the removal of bone by the osteoclasts, followed by the synthesis and mineralization of new bone matrix by the osteoblasts within the cavity created. Under normal circumstances the sequence is always that of resorption followed by formation, and the amounts of bone resorbed and formed within individual remodelling units are closely balanced. The remodelling cycle lasts for 3–6 months in the adult skeleton, most of which is occupied by the formative phase. The local coupling between resorption and formation keeps an overall constant bone mass in the adult on a week-to-week basis. Over the course of time, however, general or local influences can override this process and a low bone mass will arise if resorption exceeds formation (Figure 1.3).

The control of bone remodelling is complex, depending on both systemic and local factors and results from the interaction of

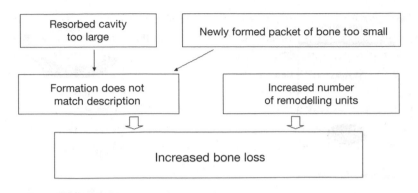

Figure 1.3 Abnormalities in osteoporosis.

mechanical stresses, systemic hormones and locally produced cytokines, prostaglandins and growth factors. Mechanical stimuli are a major determinant of the size, shape and microarchitecture of bones during skeletal growth and they subsequently play an important role in the maintenance of bone mass. The systemic calcium regulating hormones that influence bone remodelling include parathyroid hormone (PTH), calcitonin and vitamin D metabolites. PTH is a hormone synthesized by the chief cells of the parathyroid gland and it has effects on both osteoclasts and osteoblasts. In addition, physiologically PTH is the most important regulator of extracellular calcium concentration and therefore some of its effects on bone are indirect. The C cells of the thyroid gland produce calcitonin. It directly inhibits osteoclastic bone resorption and does not increase the deposition of calcium in the skeleton unless bone turnover is high. Vitamin D is hydroxylated initially by the liver and its activity is subsequently regulated in the kidney where the active metabolite 1,25-dihydroxyvitamin D is produced. It is this type of vitamin D that acts on the intestine and skeleton to maintain blood calcium supply. Other hormones that impact on the remodelling cycle include the growth hormone and sex hormones. Growth hormone plays an important part in skeletal growth, increasing bone turnover, with a net increase in bone mass and in periosteal appositional growth. Sex hormones have marked effects on the skeleton and deficiencies are associated with low bone mass in both children and adults. Oestrogens act on the skeleton via the osteoblasts that contain nuclear receptors.

Glucocorticoid receptors occur in bone cells and glucocorticoids have both direct and indirect effects on the skeleton. Whereas normal physiological concentrations play a positive role in osteoblastic function, high doses suppress osteoblastic bone formation, impair skeletal growth, decrease calcium absorption and decrease bone mass. Cytokines are locally active factors formed by immunologically competent cells. Although the effects of cytokines are not clearly understood, they appear to act both directly and indirectly on the remodelling cycle.

Bone mass throughout life

Bone mass changes throughout life in three major phases: growth, consolidation and involution. Up to 90% of the ultimate bone mass is deposited during skeletal growth, which lasts until the closure of the epiphyses. There is then a phase of skeletal consolidation lasting for up to 15 years, when bone mass increases further until the peak bone mass is achieved in the mid-30s. The peak bone mass attained is a major determinant of subsequent bone mass and fracture risk in later life. Involutional bone loss starts between the ages of 35 and 40 in both sexes, but in women there is an acceleration of bone loss in the decade after the menopause. Overall, women lose 35–50% of trabecular and 25–30% of cortical bone mass with advancing age (Figure 1.4), whereas men lose 15–45% of trabecular and 5–15% of cortical bone.

Normal woman   Osteoporotic woman

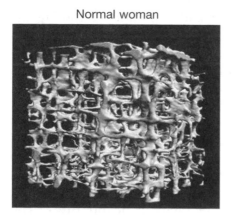 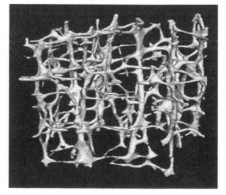

Figure 1.4 Trabecular architecture in osteoporosis. (From Borah et al. 2001.)

Bone growth

The framework of the skeleton is apparent early in fetal development with the long bones attaining their future shape and proportions by about 26 weeks. The newborn skeleton contains approximately 25 g calcium and, if this were acquired at a constant rate throughout gestation, the demand could be met from the maternal diet. Calcium demand, however, increases towards the end of pregnancy to as much as 200 mg/day. This may be in excess of the amount absorbed by the mother, and unless dietary intake or absorption efficiency increases the mother will lose calcium from her skeleton. Under normal circumstances this loss is restored after the birth of the baby.

Bones grow in size during the first two decades of life, with acceleration during adolescence, this growth phase producing about 90% of the peak bone mass attained during adult life. The most dramatic changes occur through linear growth of the long bones by alterations at the growth plate; through infancy and childhood bones expand by subperiosteal apposition and remodel by subperiosteal and endosteal resorption. Bone growth is less in girls than in boys, with girls having significantly lower bone mass than boys by 5 years of age, even after allowance for differences in height and weight. The rapid increase in bone growth in adolescence parallels the adolescent spurt in height. In boys the period of gain coincides with a steep rise in serum testosterone, suggesting a role for this hormone in the initiation of both linear growth and bone mineralization. The peak increase in bone mineralization in girls occurs at age 11–12 years, a time of rapidly increasing concentrations of oestrone and estradiol. Following the adolescent growth spurt, bone mass continues to increase by appositional growth and peak bone mass is attained during the third decade of life. The peak bone mass attained is a major determinant of subsequent bone mass and fractures in later life.

Bone loss

Bone loss starts between the ages of 35 and 40 in both sexes, with an increase in the decade following the menopause in women, as a result of a marked reduction in circulating estradiol concentrations. The onset of bone loss is likely to be genetically predetermined, with the subsequent rate of loss also being influenced by genetic factors. Although age-related bone loss occurs in both cortical and trabecular bone, its onset and rate are varied with greater losses occurring in trabecular bone as a result of its increased metabolic activity. Cortical bone loss occurs by endosteal bone resorption and increased cortical porosity, with trabecular thinning, penetration and erosion resulting in overall trabecular bone loss and loss of connectivity. Thinning occurs in both sexes whereas penetration and erosion constitute the

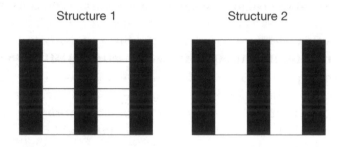

Figure 1.5 Trabecular architecture and bone strength. Assume volume 1 = volume 2 and identical material and dimensions for both. Structure 1 is 16 x stronger than structure 2. (From Bell et al. 1967.)

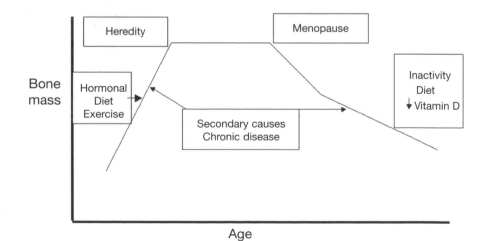

Figure 1.6 Factors affecting bone mass and bone loss.

major structural change in women. Age-related bone loss is related to increased bone turnover and an imbalance in the remodelling cycle when the amount of bone formed within individual bone remodelling units is less than that resorbed. This form of bone loss is irreversible within the remodelling unit once the remodelling cycle has been completed. The alterations in bone remodelling associated with age-related bone loss determine the accompanying changes in bone architecture (Figure 1.5), which is an important determinant of bone strength and fracture risk. Other determinants of bone strength include bone mass, geometry, composition and the balance of fatigue, micro-damage and its repair.

Factors influencing bone mass and bone loss (Figure 1.6)

Heredity

Although it is difficult to separate the roles of heredity and environment in the determination of peak bone mass, it is considered that genetic factors account for as much as 80% of the variance (Slemenda et al. 1991). The onset and subsequent rate of bone loss are also likely to be genetically predetermined. The evidence supporting the influence of heredity is provided from several different types of investigation: the study of bone mineral content in different races, twin studies comparing bone mineral density (BMD) in monozygotic and dizygotic twins, and the study of bone mineral content in families.

There are racial differences in skeletal size, with black people having larger, heavier bones and a lower fracture risk (Melton 1991). Differences in bone vertebral density become apparent in the late state of puberty but differences in cortical bone mass are present throughout childhood. Differences in bone mass alone may not fully explain the differences in fracture risk, e.g. the frequency of falling is less in black people than among white people. Twin and family studies have shown that genetic factors play an important role in regulating bone density, skeletal geometry and bone turnover as well as contributing to the pathogenesis of osteoporotic fracture itself. Some families are small boned and others large boned. Bone mass is often lower in young women whose mothers have sustained osteoporotic fractures. Most twin studies have concentrated on peak bone mass in females and have shown very consistent results with a greater concordance of bone mass between monozygotic than between dizygotic pairs (Slemenda et al. 1991). Twin studies, focusing on postmenopausal bone density, have demonstrated a continuing significant genetic component, but this is not so great, suggesting that with advancing age other factors also assume importance.

In attempting to disentangle the genetic factors underlying the risk of osteoporosis two approaches have been applied: the genome search approach and the candidate gene approach. The Human Genome Project has now identified every human gene and has uncovered many polymorphic variants of these genes that embody the genetic risk factors. The use of large-scale genome searches could indicate chromosomal areas that might contain osteoporosis genes, although this approach has not resulted in many genes being identified as osteoporosis risk genes. The candidate gene approach builds upon the known involvement of a particular gene in aspects of osteoporosis, and most of the work in the field of osteoporosis genetics has focused on candidate gene studies in populations and case–control studies. Numerous candidate genes have been tested for association and linkage with osteoporosis; however, these candidate genes are often neither essential nor sufficient to produce osteoporosis on their own. Among the most widely studied genes are the vitamin D receptor gene (*VDR*), the collagen type I α_1 gene (*COLIA1*) and the oestrogen receptor gene (*ER*). Polymorphisms of *VDR* have been associated with bone mass in several studies and there is evidence to suggest that these effects may be modified by calcium and vitamin D intake. Work on the *COLIA1* gene has suggested that this is associated with low BMD and fracture risk (Mann et al. 2001). The *ER* gene has been associated with bone density in several studies but the effects on fracture have been less widely investigated (Ralston 2002). It is likely that in the future there will be more association analyses being performed on an increasing number of candidate genes for osteoporosis.

Hormonal

Gonadal hormones are probably the most important determinants of skeletal mass in women with an association between hypogonadism and low body mass in males. A constitutional delay in puberty decreases the ultimate height of individuals. Spinal growth is more markedly impaired compared with that of the long bones, and final BMD is decreased in men and women. Although there is less evidence of the effects of pubertal timing on bone mass, size and density in men, it is generally thought that those with constitutionally delayed puberty have deficits in size, mass and bone density.

Delayed menarche, caused by either environmental factors, e.g. malnutrition, or other causes of gonadal failure, e.g. Turner's syndrome, may account for impaired low bone mass in women. In men Klinefelter's syndrome is associated with a decrease in bone mass and an increased risk of osteoporotic fractures in later life. More subtle alterations in gonadal status might alter adult bone mass. Parity and frequency of lactation have been suggested as being beneficial to the skeleton but population and retrospective studies have demonstrated disparate conclusions on these factors. The use of oral contraceptives is reported to be associated with a higher bone mass at maturity than in women who do not use oral contraceptives (Recker et al. 1992). There is, however, conflicting evidence concerning the effects of long-term progestogens on bone density. Depo-Provera is a long-acting progestogen that is commonly used. After 1 year of use, most women develop amenorrhoea and there is therefore concern over its potential effect on bone. The use of Depo-Provera is associated with an initial rapid decrease in BMD at the spine and hip, which then continues at a slower rate. On discontinuation of therapy bone mineral deficit appears to be partly reversible. In 1941 Albright and colleagues first proposed that loss of ovarian function caused increased bone loss and possible osteoporosis. These findings have been substantiated in many subsequent studies in women who have undergone both natural and surgically induced menopause. Although women are not all equally affected, bone appears to be lost most rapidly within 5 years of the menopause with a slower rate of bone loss in later postmenopausal years. In men it is now apparent that the actions of testosterone are mediated, in part, by aromatization to estradiol, such that oestrogen deficiency may also contribute to age-related bone loss in men (Riggs et al. 1998).

Nutritional

Many nutritional factors have been invoked as important for the attainment and maintenance of bone mass, including the dietary intake of protein, sodium, caffeine and alcohol. However, the greatest attention has been focused on the effect of calcium on peak bone mass. It is clearly evident that without calcium there would be impaired mineralization of the skeleton and therefore the question is not whether calcium is important, but how much is required to optimize bone mass. At birth, the skeleton contains about 25 g calcium but this increases to 1200 g in the adult with up to 400 mg calcium/day accreted into the skeleton during growth. Calcium absorption is inefficient with urinary loss and thus the large daily requirement must be maintained from dietary sources. On balance most epidemiological studies have shown that low calcium intakes during childhood and adolescence are associated with an increased risk of osteoporosis in later life. Calcium needs are greatest during adolescence with adolescents absorbing and retaining more calcium from their diets than either children or young adults. The role of calcium and its effect on bone loss remains controversial but skeletal losses after the menopause may be accelerated by low calcium diets and pharmacological doses of calcium may delay the rate of bone loss.

Prolonged vitamin D deficiency in childhood delays puberty and is likely to decrease bone mass in relation to the height attained. The relationship of this to osteoporotic fracture in later life is not known. There is a reduction in circulating 25-hydroxyvitamin D (25[OH]D) and 1,25-dihydroxy-vitamin D (1,25[OH]$_2$-D) concentrations with advancing age, resulting from decreased cutaneous production and impaired metabolism of vitamin D. This is likely to contribute to the observed increase in circulating PTH and may ultimately influence bone loss.

Other nutrients that have been suggested as potential determinants of the rate of bone loss include fluoride, protein and sodium, but their importance is still uncertain.

Bodyweight is an important determinant of bone density and fracture risk, because bone loss is more rapid in postmenopausal women with low bodyweight and individuals with osteoporotic fractures are lighter than expected. The protective effects of high bodyweight on bone density and fracture risk may be a result of the stimulation of bone formation by greater mechanical loading, increased conversion of adrenal androgens to oestrogens in fat and the shock-absorbing properties of subcutaneous fat.

Smoking may increase bone loss by reducing the age at menopause by several years, decreasing plasma oestrogen levels by increasing their metabolism, and possibly depressing osteoblast function. The deleterious effect of smoking on the skeleton may also result in part from the association with low bodyweight. Although alcoholism is a recognized cause of osteoporosis, the effect of modest alcohol consumption on bone density remains unclear.

Activity

Physical activity is important to the skeleton because the associated weight-bearing and muscular activity stimulate bone formation and increase bone mass, whereas immobilization leads to rapid bone loss. The positive responses of the skeleton to physical activity are site specific to the loading pattern, and the type of activity also influences the degree of response of the bone to loading. Numerous studies have reported the positive effects in adults and children of various types of exercise, ranging from repetitive strength training to recreational gymnastics (Bassey 2001). The decline in physical activity with advancing age is likely to cause bone loss and, as there is already an imbalance between formation and resorption, skeletal losses can be considerably accelerated.

Our understanding of osteoporosis depends upon clear definition of the cellular, biochemical, mechanical and epidemiological features of bone growth and involution. At the cellular level, the skeleton must be viewed as a dynamic organ undergoing cyclical remodelling through the actions of its constituent cells. At the biochemical level, increasing awareness is focused on the structure and properties of bone matrix. The biomechanical properties of bone tissue and the contribution of non-mineral bony elements to its strength are also important. The concepts of bone mass and bone loss, determined by a combination of genetic potential, diet, exercise and hormonal status, are also central to the pathogenesis and subsequent management of osteoporosis.

References

Albright F, Smith PH, Richardson AM (1941) Postmenopausal osteoporosis. Its clinical features. JAMA 116: 2465–74.

Bassey EJ (2001) Exercise for improving bone mineral density: The benefits of weight training. Osteopor Rev 9(4): 11–13.

Bell GM, Dunbar O, Beck JS, Gibb A (1967) Variations in strength of vertebrae with age and their relationship to osteoporosis. Calcif Tissue Res 1: 75–86.

Borah B, Gross GJ, Dufresne TE et al. (2001) Three-dimensional micro-imaging (MRmicro I and micro CT) finite element modelling and rapid prototyping provide insights into bone architecture in osteoporosis. Anat Rec 265: 101–10.

Lanyon LE (1992) The success and failure of the adaptive response to functional load bearing in averting vertebral fracture. Bone 13(suppl 2): S17–21

Mann V, Hobson EE, Li B et al. (2001) A COLIA1 Sp 1 binding site polymorphism predisposes to osteoporotic fracture by affecting bone density and quality. J Clin Invest 107: 899–907.

Melton LJ (1991) Differing patterns of osteoporosis across the world. In: Chesnut CH III (ed.), New Dimensions in the 1990s. Hong Kong: Excerpta Medica Asia, pp. 13–18.

Owen ME (1985) Lineage of osteogenic cells and their relationship to the stromal system. In: Peck WA (ed.), Bone and Mineral Research, Vol. 3. Amsterdam: Elsevier, pp. 1–25.

Ralston SH (2002) Genetics of complex diseases: The bad and the good genes. Osteopor Int 13(suppl 1): S2.

Recker RR, Davies M, Hinders M et al. (1992) Bone gain in young adults. JAMA 268: 2403–8.

Riggs BL, Khosla S, Melton LJ III (1998) A unitary model for involutional osteoporosis: Oestrogen deficiency causes both type I and type II osteoporosis and contributes to bone loss in ageing men. J Bone Miner Res 13: 763–73.

Slemenda CW, Christian JC, Williams CJ, Norton JA, Johnston CCL (1991) Genetic determinants of bone mass in adult women: A reevaluation of the twin model and the potential importance of gene interaction on heritability estimates. J Bone Miner Res 6: 561–7.

Suda T, Takahoshi N, Martin TJ (1992) Modulation of osteoclast differentiation. Endocr Rev 13: 66–80.

CHAPTER 2
Secondary osteoporosis

- There are numerous causes of secondary osteoporosis
- In some studies, 20–30% of postmenopausal women and more than 50% of men with osteoporosis are found to have an underlying cause
- It is important that medical disorders are recognized and appropriate interventions are undertaken in the management of secondary osteoporosis

Secondary osteoporosis is defined as bone loss that results from specific, well-defined clinical disorders, which are highlighted in this chapter. This large and diverse group includes adverse effects of medications, endocrine abnormalities, disorders of the gastrointestinal or biliary tract, immobilization, renal disease and cancer. It is difficult to ascertain the true incidence of secondary osteoporosis but several studies have estimated that it may occur in 20–30% of postmenopausal women and in more than 50% of men with osteoporosis (Caplan et al. 1994, Kelepouris et al. 1995). Many times secondary causes are not considered in a patient with low bone mineral density (BMD) but often the adverse effects of osteoporosis are reversible with appropriate intervention. Detailed history taking should help to elicit underlying secondary causes and routine investigations may highlight previously undiagnosed conditions.

Secondary osteoporosis associated with drug therapy

Causes of secondary osteoporosis: drugs

- Glucocorticoids
- Anticonvulsants
- Heparin
- ? Methotrexate

Glucocorticoid-induced osteoporosis

Glucocorticoids are used to treat a wide variety of medical conditions and at any one time about 1% of the adult population in UK is taking oral glucocorticoids, with this figure increasing to 2.4% in the eighth decade of life.

Glucocorticoid-induced osteoporosis (GIOP) was discovered more than 60 years ago when Cushing (1932) first described the tendency of patients with excess endogenous glucocorticoids to develop fractures. The relevance of these findings to exogenous oral glucocorticoids remained controversial for some time but the importance of this type of osteoporosis has now been well established.

Glucocorticoids affect bone through multiple pathways, inhibiting osteoblast proliferation and stimulating osteoclast function. They also decrease calcium absorption and increase urinary phosphate and calcium loss by direct effects on the kidney. In turn these two mechanisms lead to secondary hyperparathyroidism and hence to increased bone resorption. As glucocorticoids also influence the production and action of many hormones, cytokines and growth factors that regulate bone and calcium metabolism, some of their effects may be indirect. Many cross-sectional studies have found that patients using oral glucocorticoids have reduced BMD and increased risk of fracture. This risk, independent of underlying disease, age and gender, increases rapidly after the start of therapy (within 3–6 months) and decreases within about 1 year of stopping therapy. The General Practice Research Database (GPRD) study (Van Staa et al. 2000) conducted in primary care in the UK has evaluated fracture incidence in

244 235 users of glucocorticoids. This study confirmed rapid onset of both vertebral and non-vertebral fractures after starting therapy. It also found a strong relationship between daily dose and risk of fracture, with those patients on a daily dose of 20 mg prednisolone having a 60% higher rate of non-vertebral fractures than control cases. In addition cumulative dose of glucocorticoids was also associated with an increased risk of fracture.

Although oral glucocorticoids are known to increase the risk of fracture in adults their effects in children remain uncertain. More than 1% of the children in the UK receive a course of glucocorticoid therapy during any 1-year period. A study of 37 562 children showed that they mostly received the high dose for a short period of time. Sporadic use of high doses was not associated with an increased risk of fracture in children and once treatment was stopped risk of fracture was minimal. However, children who used glucocorticoids regularly had an increased risk of fracture and it is this group that merits particular attention (Van Staa et al. 2003). One of the major concerns with gluco-corticoid use in children is that peak bone mass will be below normal as a result of the inhibition of bone formation. Peak BMD is a strong predictor of fracture risk in later life and consequently childhood use of glucocorticoids may result in increased fracture risk in later life.

Estimates indicate that there are about a million adult users of inhaled glucocorticoids in the UK (Lipworth 1999) and there is now increasing concern about the potential systematic effects of long-term use of inhaled steroids. A Cochrane meta-analysis of seven randomized trials of patients, mostly aged under 60, did not suggest an increased risk of fracture or excess bone loss when inhaled steroids were used for fewer than 3 years (Jones et al. 2003). This study does not, how-ever, address the long-term effects of inhaled glucocorticoids in elderly patients or in patients with severe respiratory disease. A further large meta-analysis in 2003 (Richy et al. 2003) showed that many stud-ies demonstrated that inhaled glucocorticoid therapy resulted in lower BMD and dose-related increases in fracture risk. It is, however, unclear whether or not this increased risk is directly related to therapy or to underlying disease.

General measures to reduce bone loss include minimizing the dose of glucocorticoids, considering alternative formulations or routes of admin-istration, and prescribing alternative immunosuppressive agents. Good nutrition, an adequate dietary calcium intake and physical activity should be encouraged, and tobacco use and alcohol abuse avoided. In an attempt to improve the management of GIOP, evidence-based guidelines were produced by the Royal College of Physicians in collaboration with the Bone and Tooth Society and the National Osteoporosis Society in 2002 (RCP 2002) (Figure 2.1). These guidelines suggest that those aged over 65 or those with a prior fragility fracture, and receiving oral prednisolone for at least 3 months, should be advised to start bone-protective therapy at the time of starting glucocorticoids. In younger individuals, BMD measurements should be considered to inform treatment decisions. A T score of -1.5 or lower may indicate the need for intervention (T score is the bone density value expressed in standard deviation units with reference to the young normal range consisting of individuals at peak bone mass), but the effect of age on individual fracture risk should be taken into account. These guidelines do not address the question of whether patients who frequently receive short doses of glucocorticoids or use regular inhaled steroids need BMD monitoring and/or treatment.

Anticonvulsant medications

Bone disease associated with anticonvulsant therapy is a form of osteomalacia and in this condition high-turnover osteoporosis is often present. The mechanism by which phenobarbitone and carbamazepine induce bone loss is possibly the increased metabolism and clearance of vitamin D by the liver. Anticonvulsants such as sodium valproate have little or no impact on serum calcium and 25-hydroxyvitamin D levels because they do not induce hepatic drug metabolites and enzymes.

Miscellaneous medications

Methotrexate has been implicated as a cause of bone loss, but, in most studies, other drugs have been administered or the gonadal status of the patients has been altered, making definitive conclusions difficult. Heparin has been implicated in the suppression of bone formation. Bile acid-binding resins, such as cholestyramine, have the potential to interfere with vitamin D absorption.

MANAGEMENT OF GLUCOCORTICOID INDUCE DOSTEOPOROSIS

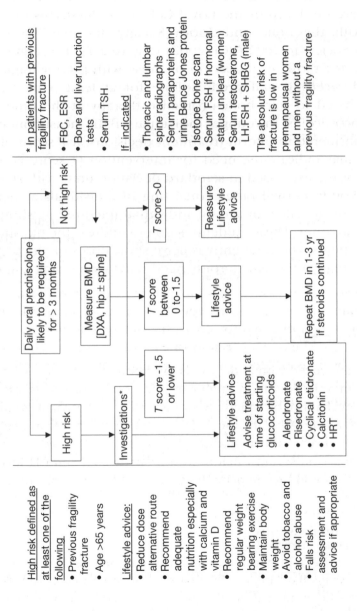

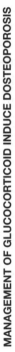

Figure 2.1 Management of glucocorticoid-induced osteoporosis. BMD, bone mineral density; DXA, dual energy X-ray absorptiometry; ESR, erythrocyte sedimentation rate; FBC, full blood count; FSH, follicle-stimulating hormone; HRT, hormone replacement therapy; LH, luteinizing hormone; SHBG, sex hormone-binding globulin; TSH, thyroid-stimulating hormone. (Adapted from the guidelines of Royal College of Physicians of London and Bone and Tooth Society of Great Britain 2000.)

Endocrine disorders associated with secondary osteoporosis

Causes of secondary osteoporosis: endocrine

* Hyperthyroidism
* Hyperparathyroidism
* Diabetes
* Male hypogonadism
* Hyperprolactinaemia

Hyperthyroidism

In the thyrotoxic patient with excessive levels of thyroid hormone, the bone-remodelling cycle is shortened, leading to a decrease in bone formation with an overall failure to replace resorbed bone completely and consequent bone loss. Several studies have indicated that individuals with a history of thyrotoxicosis have an increased risk of fracture and may sustain fracture at an early age (Cummings et al. 1995). After effective treatment of the thyrotoxicosis, the decrease in bone density may be reversible. The administration of excessive exogenous thyroid hormone has been associated with osteopenia. However, the clinical relevance of osteoporosis associated with iatrogenic hyperthyroidism has been examined in terms of the development of fractures, although the data remain controversial. There are concerns about the effects of administration of high doses of thyroid hormone to suppress thyrotrophin secretion in patients with differentiated thyroid cancer or non-toxic goitre. It is possible that, in patients who have other risk factors for osteoporosis, this type of therapy may aggravate fracture risk (Obermayer-Pietsch et al. 2000).

Primary hyperparathyroidism

Primary hyperparathyroidism is usually asymptomatic and is a common disorder, with an incidence of 1 in 500 to 1 in 1000 (Bilezikian and Silverberg 2000). Parathyroid hormone (PTH) is responsible for maintaining calcium homoeostasis through its action on target cells in the bone and kidney. In primary hyperparathyroidism, the parathyroid cell loses its normal sensitivity to calcium, which leads to a decline in the normal feedback control of PTH by extracellular calcium. As a result there is an increase in circulating levels of PTH associated with increased bone turnover, leading to an eventual loss in both trabecular and cortical bones. Several studies have assessed the risk of fracture in patients with primary hyperparathyroidism and these have shown an increased incidence of vertebral, Colles', rib and pelvic fractures (Vestergaard et al. 2000). With marked hyperparathyroidism, surgical intervention will be necessary, usually with excellent results. BMD improves spontaneously in both the forearm and the lumbar spine with rapid increases seen within a year.

Diabetes mellitus

Low BMD is associated with type 1 diabetes mellitus, although the mechanisms of bone loss remain controversial. No increase in the incidence of fracture has been noted in patients who have diabetes with the exception of stress fractures in foot bones (Leidig-Bruckner and Ziegler 2001).

Male hypogonadism

Hypogonadism is a well-established cause of osteoporosis in males, occurring in up to 20% of men with vertebral crush fractures and 50% of elderly men with hip fractures. Causes of hypogonadal osteoporosis in men include Klinefelter syndrome, idiopathic hypogonadotrophic hypogonadism, hyperprolactinaemia, haemochromatosis and primary testicular failure. Studies have shown an increased bone resorption and decreased mineralization, which has been attributed to androgen and oestrogen deficiency, low vitamin D concentrations and malabsorption of calcium. These abnormalities may be reversed by treatment with testosterone, leading to an increase in BMD (Behre et al. 1999). The diagnosis of hypogonadism may not always be clinically apparent in men with osteoporosis, so routine measurement of serum testosterone and gonadotrophins is probably worth while (Scane and Francis 1993).

Hyperprolactinaemia

Hyperprolactinaemia occurs in physiological conditions such as pregnancy and lactation and also secondary to pituitary or hypothalamic diseases. It has been estimated that as many as 25–30% of pre-menopausal women with amenorrhoea may have hyperprolactinaemia, which in turn is associated with reduced bone mass (Biller et al. 1992). Both men and women with a history of prolactinaemia and hypogo-nadism for more than 10 years have lower BMD levels, suggesting that the severity of bone loss is related to the presence and duration of hypog-onadism. Treatment of hyperprolactinaemia with either bromocriptine or surgery increases bone density, but only partially corrects the osteo-porosis.

Osteoporosis associated with gastrointestinal, pancreatic and hepatic disorders

The skeleton depends on the adequate supply of calcium, phosphate and vitamin D from the diet. Gastrointestinal disease leads to abnor-malities in bone as a result of the malabsorption of vitamin D and calcium, although the presence of the disease itself may lead to reduced intake or limited exposure to sunlight. In addition protein and other micronutrient deficiencies may contribute to bone loss in gastrointestinal tract disorders.

Causes of secondary osteoporosis: gastrointestinal conditions

- Gastric surgery
- Coeliac disease
- Inflammatory bowel disease
- Liver disease

Osteoporosis, pseudofractures and fractures have been noted in patients after gastrectomy with females being more prone to develop these, possibly several years after surgery. Possible factors in the patho-genesis of bone loss after gastric surgery include decreased absorption of vitamin D, malabsorption of calcium, the absence of gastric acid and intestinal hurry, and the reduced food intake that commonly follows gastric surgery.

Coeliac disease

Bone disease with coeliac disease can present as osteoporosis or osteomalacia or both. Untreated adults usually present with reduced BMD at the time of diagnosis whereas children may present with growth retardation (Meyer et al. 2001). Patients may present with normal serum biochemical analysis or with reduced serum and urine calcium levels and elevated alkaline phosphatase levels. With a gluten-free diet, biochemical abnormalities and BMD measurements may improve (Kemppainen et al. 1999).

Inflammatory bowel disease

Bone disease can be associated with inflammatory bowel disease, such as Crohn's disease or ulcerative colitis. Skeletal bone disease is most frequently associated with Crohn's disease, especially if treated with ileal resection and glucocorticoids. In a study by Schulte et al. (1998), the incidence of osteopenia was 32% in patients with ulcerative colitis and 36% in those with Crohn's disease, with the incidence of osteoporosis being 7% and 15% respectively. In Crohn's disease there are multiple reasons for the development of bone disease because malabsorption results in the reduction of vitamin D and calcium absorption; steatorrhoea may also occur causing a decrease in calcium and vitamin D absorption.

Diseases of the liver

Liver disease may lead to osteoporosis because of the inability of the liver to convert vitamin D to 25-hydroxyvitamin D and also because of the liver's inability to transport vitamin D metabolites to the target tissues.

Alcohol abuse is a major cause of liver disease with cirrhosis contributing to the severity of bone disease. Vertebral osteopenia may be observed in up to 50% of ambulatory patients, with alcoholism and fractures of the ribs and vertebrae occurring in 30% of this population. Chronic alcohol abuse has a detrimental effect on the male skeleton, whereas a neutral or beneficial effect with light-to-moderate alcohol consumption is seen on the female skeleton (Turner 2000). Alcohol directly inhibits bone cell activity, resulting in reduced bone formation and resorption. Other possible causes of bone loss in alcoholism include poor diet, malabsorption of calcium as a result of vitamin D deficiency, alcohol-induced loss of calcium in the urine and alcohol-related liver disease.

Transplantation osteoporosis

Organ transplantation has become an effective therapy for end-stage renal, hepatic, cardiac and pulmonary disease. One-year patient survival is excellent and many patients now live for more than 10 years. Unfortunately many patients demonstrate a propensity to fracture, which greatly impacts on their quality of life. The pathogenesis of this type of osteoporosis is not completely understood but risk factors include white race, older age, postmenopausal status, vitamin D and dietary calcium deficiency, and excessive use of tobacco and alcohol. In addition transplant recipients are exposed to a number of drugs implicated in bone loss, e.g. glucocorticoids and immunosuppressants. After renal transplantation it is estimated that there will be excess spine bone loss of 3–6% in the first 6 months, with a fracture prevalence ranging from 7% to 11% (Horber et al. 1994). After cardiac transplantation lumbar spine BMD decreases by 6–10% in the first 6 months and thereafter appears to stabilize. A longitudinal study demonstrated that 36% of patients sustained one or more fractures during the first year after transplantation, despite treatment with calcium and cholecalciferol (Shane et al. 1997). Prior glucocorticoid therapy, tobacco use and hypoxaemia may be associated with pre-transplantation osteoporosis in patients with lung disease, with high fracture prevalence both before and after surgery. Before organ transplantation, it is important to measure BMD of the spine and hip because a low BMD will be associated with an increased risk of fracture. As waiting time for a transplantation may be long, aggressive treatment with an anti-resorptive agent may result in significant improvement in bone mass before transplantation (Rodino and Shane 1998). As bone loss occurs most rapidly in the first 3–6 months after transplantation and fragility fractures occur within this period, preventive strategies should be initiated immediately. Several studies have suggested that bisphosphonates may be useful at this time (Saag et al. 1998, Arlen et al. 2001), and calcitonin has also been used successfully to treat transplant-associated osteoporosis (Valero et al. 1995).

Miscellaneous causes

Anorexia nervosa and bulimia affect 5–10% of women (Nielsen 2001) with the onset being at any time from adolescence through the fourth decade of life. These eating disorders may be resistant to treatment and chronic in nature, which results in significant morbidity and mortality. It has been estimated that 50% of anorexic patients have bone density values of the lumbar spine that are more than two standard deviations below those of age-matched, healthy controls (Biller et al. 1989). There are several metabolic disorders associated with anorexia nervosa that may adversely affect the skeleton. These include oestrogen deficiency, endogenous cortisol excess, protein–energy malnutrition, and secondary hyperparathyroidism caused by low dietary calcium intake or vitamin D deficiency. Unfortunately diagnosis and treatment may be difficult, because patients are often resistant to seeking medical help and treatment.

Causes of secondary osteoporosis: other conditions

- Multiple myeloma
- Skeletal metastases
- Eating disorders
- Osteogenesis imperfecta

Cancellous and endocortical bone surfaces are in close apposition to the bone marrow and therefore disorders of bone marrow can produce profound changes in bone. Plasma cell dyscrasia, such as multiple myeloma, leukaemia and lymphomas, can all result in osteoporosis.

It is of particular note that underlying secondary causes can contribute to the development of osteoporosis and subsequent fractures. Although the large number of conditions that may predispose to secondary osteoporosis are well managed in different specialities, it is important to recognize any additional problems that the patient may have with respect to fractures should osteoporosis remain undiagnosed and untreated.

References

Arlen DJ, Lambert K, Ionnidis G, Adachi JD (2001) Treatment of established bone loss after transplantation. Transplantation 71: 669–773.

Behre HM, von Eckardstein S, Kliesch S, Niescchlag E (1999) Long term substitution therapy of hypogonadal men with transscrotal testosterone over 7–10 years. Clin Endocrinol 50: 629–35.

Bilezikian JP, Silverberg SJ (2000) Clinical spectrum of primary hyperparathyroidism. Rev Endocr Metab Disord 1: 237–45.

Biller BM, Saxe V, Herzog DB, Rosenthal DI, Holzman S, Klibanski A (1989) Mechanisms of osteoporosis in adult and adolescent women with anorexia nervosa. J Clin Endocrinol Metab 68: 548–54.

Biller BM, Baum HB, Rosenthal DI, Saxe VC, Charpie PM, Klibanski A (1992) A progressive trabecular osteopenia in women with hyperprolactinemic amenorrhea. J Clin Endocrinol Metab 75: 692–7.

Caplan GA, Scane AC, Francis RM (1994) Pathogenesis of crush fractures in women. J R Soc Med 87: 200–2.

Cummings SR, Nevitt MC, Browner WS et al. for the Study of Osteoporotic Fractures Research Group (1995) Risk factors for hip fracture in white women. N Engl J Med 332: 767–73.

Cushing H (1932) The basophilic adenomas of the pituitary body and their clinical manifestations (pituitary basophilism). Bull Johns Hopkins Hosp 1: 137–92

Horber FF, Casez JP, Steiger U, Czerniak A, Montandon A, Jaeger P (1994) Changes in bone mass early after kidney transplantation. J Bone Miner Res 9: 1–9.

Jones A, Fay JK, Burr M, Stone M, Hood K, Roberts G (2003) Inhaled corticosteroid effects on bone metabolism and mild chronic obstructive pulmonary diseases (Cochrane Review). The Cochrane Library, Issue 3. Oxford: Update Software.

Kelepouris N, Harper KD, Gannon F, Kaplan FS, Haddad JG (1995) Severe osteoporosis in men. Ann Intern Med 123: 452–60.

Kemppainen T, Kroger H, Janatuinen E et al. (1999) Effect of gluten free diet: A 5 year follow up study. Bone 25: 355–60.

Leidig-Bruckner G, Ziegler R (2001) Diabetes Mellitus a risk for osteoporosis? Exp Clin Endocrinol Diabetes 109(suppl 2): S493–514.

Lipworth BJ (1999) Systemic adverse effects of inhaled corticosteroid therapy: A systematic review and meta-analysis. Arch Intern Med 159: 941–55.

Meyer D, Stavropolous S, Diamond B, Shane E, Green PH (2001) Osteoporosis in a North American adult population with coeliac disease. Am J Gastroenterol 96: 112–19.

Nielsen S (2001) Epidemiology and mortality of eating disorders. Psychiatr Clin North Am 24: 201–14.

Obermayer-Pietsch B, Dobnig H, Warmkoss H et al. (2000) Variable bone mass recovery in hyperthyroid bone disease after radioiodine therapy in post menopausal patients. Maturitas 35: 159–66.

Richy F, Bousquet J, Ehrlich GE et al. (2003) Inhaled corticosteroids, effects on bone in asthmatic and COPD patients: a quantitative systematic review. Osteopor Int 14: 179–90.

Rodino MA, Shane E (1998) Osteoporosis after organ transplantation. Am J Med 104: 459–69.

Royal College of Physicians (2002) Glucocorticoid Induced Osteoporosis: Guidelines for prevention and treatment. London: Royal College of Physicians.

Royal College of Physicians of London and Bone and Tooth Society of Great Britain (2000) Clinical Guidelines for Prevention and Treatment. London: Royal College of Physicians.

Saag KG, Emkey R, Schnitzer TJ et al. (1998) Alendronate for the prevention and treatment of glucocorticoid osteoporosis. N Engl J Med 339: 292–9.

Scane AC, Francis RM (1993) Risk factors for osteoporosis in men. Clin Endocrinol 38: 15–16.

Schulte C, Dignass AU, Mann K, Goebell H (1998) Reduced bone mineral density and unbalanced bone metabolism in patients with inflammatory bowel disease. Inflam Bowel Dis 4: 268–75.

Shane E, Rivas M, McMahon DJ et al. (1997) Bone loss and turnover after cardiac transplantation. J Clin Endocrinol Metab 82: 1497–506.

Turner RT (2000) Skeletal response to alcohol. Alcohol Clin Exp Res 24: 1693–701.

Valero MA, Loinaz C, Larrodera L, Leon M, Moreno E, Hawkins F (1995) Calcitonin and bisphosphonates treatment in bone loss after liver transplantation. Calcif Tissue Int 57: 15–19.

Van Staa TP, Leufkens HGM, Abenhaim, L, Zhang B, Cooper C (2000) Fracture and oral corticosteroids: Relationship to daily and cumulative dose. Rheumatology (Oxford) 39: 1383–9.

Van Staa TP, Cooper C, Leufkens HGM, Bishop N (2003) Children and the risk of fractures caused by oral corticosteroids. J Bone Miner Res 18: 913–18.

Vestergaard P, Mollerup CL, Frokjaer VG, Christiansen P, Blicher-Toft M, Mosekilde L (2000) Cohort study of risk of fracture before and after surgery for primary hyperparathyroidism. BMJ 321: 598–602.

CHAPTER 3
Osteoporosis and fractures

- In osteoporosis there is a lower bone mass than expected and an increased risk of fractures
- Fractures at the spine and hip are common and cause excess mortality and morbidity
- Fracture incidence is influenced by both skeletal and non-skeletal factors
- Management includes early surgery, if appropriate, pain relief and prevention of further fractures
- Management of falls is closely linked to fracture prevention

The adverse outcomes of osteoporosis relate mainly to osteoporotic fractures. Hip and spine fractures are linked to increased mortality and all fractures may lead to disability and reduced quality of life. This chapter reviews overall epidemiology of fractures and determinants of fracture risk, and discusses specific management of spine and hip fractures. It also covers the relationship between falls and fractures, and the relevance of falls prevention.

Osteoporosis has been internationally defined as:

> A progressive systemic skeletal disease characterised by low bone mass and micro-architectural deterioration of bone tissue, with a consequent increase in bone fragility and susceptibility to fracture.
>
> World Health Organization (WHO 1994)

From a quantitative perspective, the WHO has, in addition, recommended thresholds of bone mineral density (BMD) in women that may also be used to define osteoporosis; these have been widely, but not universally, accepted by the international scientific community and regulatory agencies. Using this method, osteoporosis in postmenopausal white women is defined as a value of BMD that is more than 2.5 standard deviations (SDs) below the young average value. Severe osteoporosis uses the same threshold but also includes the presence of one or more fragility fractures.

Osteoporotic fractures

In the UK, there are 180,000 fractures each year, including 41,000 forearm, 25,000 vertebral and 70,000 hip fractures.

Excess mortality and substantial morbidity after hip fractures and symptomatic vertebral fractures.

Annual cost of osteoporotic fractures in the UK has been estimated at £1.7 billion.

Eastell et al. (2001, p. 575)

The term 'osteoporosis' was first used in the nineteenth century as a histological description for aged bone tissue, but its clinical consequences were not appreciated until 150 years ago when Sir Astley Cooper recognized that hip fractures might result from an age-related reduction in bone mass or quality. In the UK osteoporosis results in over 200 000 fractures per year with the most common ones occurring at the forearm, vertebral body and femoral neck; in addition, fractures of the humerus, tibia, pelvis and ribs are common in those with osteoporosis. The likelihood that any individual will have an osteoporotic fracture is relatively high. In the UK, in women the lifetime fracture incidence rates are 14%, 11% and 13% at hip, spine and forearm, respectively, whereas for men the corresponding figures are 3%, 2% and 2% (Dennison and Cooper 1996). It has been estimated that the cost of treating osteoporotic fractures in the female population alone was approximately £1.5–1.8 billion in the UK in 2000 (Torgerson 2000). The key components of these costs are attributable to hip fractures and the subsequent nursing home care that is required for a proportion of these patients. With an ageing population and increase in fracture incidence, it is estimated that costs may increase to £2.1 billion per year by 2010 (Burge et al. 2001).

Osteoporotic fractures occurring at the spine and forearm are associated with significant morbidity but the most serious consequences arise in patients with hip fracture, with a significant increase in mortality of 15–20%, particularly in elderly women and men.

Determinants of fracture risk

The risk of fracture (Figure 3.1) will be determined by the intrinsic strength of the skeletal structure, which in turn comprises BMD, bone quality, bone size, skeletal geometry and previous fracture. In addition non-skeletal factors, e.g. age and the propensity to fall, will also play a significant role in determining fracture risk. The organic matrix of bone is impregnated with mineral salts, which confer the skeleton with its properties of hardness and rigidity. The breaking strength of bone is related to its mineral content and thus it is reasonable to assume that individuals who have greater bone density are less likely to have fractures.

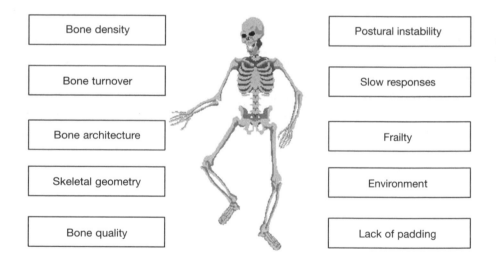

Figure 3.1 Risk of fracture.

As BMD can be practically measured with marked precision and sensitivity, the evaluation of BMD is the most commonly used method for predicting fracture risk in humans. There is a strong inverse relationship between bone density and fracture risk: the lower the bone density, the higher the risk of fracture. The strength of bone is also related to its internal architecture and quality. Structural and qualitative abnormalities that contribute to the loss of skeletal strength include changes in the turnover of bone to repair fatigue damage and the loss of connectivity of the trabecular elements comprising cancellous bone. It is possible to use biochemical measurements to assess the structural integrity and quality of bone, and recent studies have suggested that these may be independent measures of bone density loss and future fracture risk (Delmas et al. 2000). Bone size is also an important determinant of osteoporotic fractures. There is a positive relationship between body height and hip fracture, and it has been suggested that the trend towards increased body height in developed countries may be one of the factors explaining the decrease in the incidence of hip fracture. Similarly, an increase in hip axis length is associated with increased hip fracture risk independent of BMD (Faulkner et al. 1995).

Numerous studies have cited the relationship with the increased risk of further fracture after one fracture. Estimates vary on the magnitude of this, but Chaapurlat and colleagues (2003) reported a fourfold greater risk of second hip fracture after a first hip fracture. Women with one pre-existing vertebral deformity have a fivefold greater risk of further vertebral fractures (Black et al. 1999). Determinants of fracture risk also include non-skeletal risk factors, particularly age, postural instability, physical and mental frailty, and conditions associated with the risk of falling (Cummings et al. 1995).

Vertebral fractures

Symptomatic vertebral fractures are associated with significant morbidity, excess mortality, and health and social service expenditure. Vertebral fractures commonly present in the lower thoracic or upper lumbar spine and can occur spontaneously or as a result of minimal trauma such as coughing. They are classified as a central, crush or wedge fracture, with wedging being more common at the anterior than the posterior aspect of the vertebra. The major consequences of vertebral fracture are acute and potential chronic pain, with additional possible features of height loss and thoracic kyphosis.

Vertebral fractures
- Back pain
- Loss of height

- Kyphosis
- Impaired mobility
- Respiratory and digestive problems
- Lead to 15 additional GP visits per year
- Increased mortality rate of up to 30%
- Risk of another fracture within a year of 19.2%
- Risk of hip fracture increased three- to eightfold

Epidemiology

It has been difficult to quantify accurately the incidence and prevalence of vertebral fractures, because many patients with back pain do not seek medical attention (Cooper 1993). In addition, in the past there has been a lack of a universally recognized definition of vertebral deformity from radiographs of the spine. However, the lifetime risk of symptomatic fracture for a 30-year-old white woman in the UK has been calculated to be 11%, compared with 2% for a man of the same age. A large epidemiological study conducted throughout Europe, the European Vertebral Osteoporosis Study (EVOS), showed that the overall prevalence of vertebral deformity increased in women from 5% at the age of 50 years to 25% at 75 years, whereas the corresponding figures for men were 10% and 18% (O'Neill et al. 1996). There was substantial geographical variation, with the highest rates observed in Scandinavian countries, reflecting differences in physical activity and other lifestyle factors. It has been estimated that the acute cost of vertebral fractures in the UK is £12 million per year (Torgerson 2000), although the real cost may be substantially higher than this because of the associated long-term morbidity. Patients with symptomatic vertebral fracture consult their GPs 14 times more than control individuals in the year after a fracture (Kado et al. 1999), so they are likely to continue to use health and social service resources at an increased rate.

Risk factors

There is a strong inverse relationship between bone density and risk of vertebral fractures, with the age-adjusted risk of fracture doubling with each standard deviation reduction in BMD (Van der Klift et al. 2002).

It is well documented that a prevalent osteoporotic fracture increases the risk of further fractures. The Study of Osteoporosis Fractures (SOF), a prospective study of 9704 American women aged 65 years or older, studied the relationship between prevalent vertebral deformity and further vertebral fracture (Black et al. 1999). The findings suggested that pre-existing vertebral deformity was associated with a fivefold greater risk of further vertebral fracture. In women with a previous vertebral fracture, the risk of hip fracture was also increased 2.8-fold. In 2003, Roy and colleagues showed broadly comparable values for the incidence of subsequent fractures, but this was less pronounced in men than in women.

Cross-sectional studies have examined the relationship between other putative risk factors and prevalent vertebral fractures. The risk of vertebral deformity among men was significantly elevated in those with very high levels of physical activity (Silman et al. 1997), suggesting the significance of trauma. In women, the risk of fracture was elevated in those with a late menarche, whereas advanced menopausal age was associated with a reduced risk of deformity; the use of the oral contraceptive pill was also protective (O'Neill et al. 1996). The European Prospective Osteoporosis Study (EPOS) demonstrated a trend for lower risk of incident vertebral fractures with higher weight and body mass index (BMI) in both sexes, but this was significant for BMI in men only using qualitative assessment of vertebral fracture. In this study none of the lifestyle factors, including smoking, alcohol intake, physical inactivity or milk consumption, showed a consistent association with incident vertebral fractures in either sex (Roy et al. 2003).

In about a third of women and half of men with symptomatic vertebral crush factors, there is an underlying cause of secondary osteoporosis, including oral steroid use, hypogonadism in men, alcohol abuse, hyperthyroidism, skeletal metastases and multiple myeloma (Caplan et al. 1994).

Consequences of vertebral fracture

Vertebral fractures result in significant morbidity with reductions in both physical and mental capacities, leading to a reduction in quality of life. There is also an increased mortality associated with vertebral crush fractures of about 18% at 5 years, although this may be associated with coexisting conditions rather than the actual fracture (Cooper 1993).

The consequences of vertebral fracture include back pain, kyphosis and height loss. New crush fractures may occur during everyday activities such as bending or lifting, and can give rise to severe pain of recent onset. Pain is felt at the specific site of the fracture but may also be referred around the body in a symmetrical fashion and can mimic chest or abdominal discomfort. The acute episode may be so severe that it is accompanied by shock, pallor and vomiting, with the pain being exacerbated by coughing or sneezing. This acute pain may be accompanied by paravertebral spasm and can persist for several weeks before gradually settling; during this time back movements, particularly flexion, may be limited. An uncertain proportion of patients may be left with chronic residual pain but O'Neill and colleagues (2004) have shown that there is no significant increase in the frequency of back pain for 5 years after the initial fracture, provided that no further fractures have been sustained. Chronic pain and kyphotic posture can develop insidiously as a result of vertebral microfractures. The ligamentous structures of the spine contain pain fibres and the persistent stretching is perceived as pain. The kyphotic deformity associated with osteoporosis, and the resulting iliocostal friction syndrome, is painful and interferes with normal activities. In some instances the patient does not give a history of acute pain but may present with height loss and kyphosis alone, with the fracture being diagnosed only after a radiograph has been taken.

When a thoracic kyphosis is marked, it requires the patient to hyperextend the neck and may give rise to neck pain and muscle fatigue, resulting in the chin habitually resting on the sternum. A kyphosis also reduces the thoracic volume, impairing total lung volume and, if there is coexisting lung disease, the resulting loss of vital capacity will increase breathlessness and the possibility of chest infections. As the thoracic cage descends, it may impact on the brim of the pelvis, causing pain and discomfort. In addition the resulting cosmetic effect on the body leads to problems with fitting clothes. A kyphosis may also lead to a reduction in abdominal volume, causing protrusion and digestive problems related to acid reflux and the development of a hiatus hernia.

Although pain usually decreases after a fracture there is evidence to suggest that functional impairment continues. The use of various quality-of-life measures has indicated a substantial reduction in quality of life that is comparable with other major diseases. Hall and colleagues used the Barthel and Short-form SF-36 questionnaires and demonstrated significant reductions both in functionality and in physical and mental domains of quality in life (Hall et al. 1999). Among those with fractures there was no association between quality of life or functional ability and time since fracture (mean 5.1 years), suggesting that these adverse outcomes persisted. Results from a clinic-based study in Germany demonstrated a lower degree of well-being in women with recent vertebral fractures (< 2 years) compared with those with older fractures (> 2 years); however, limitations in everyday life were similar in the two groups, suggesting that these persisted after fracture (Begerow et al. 1999). Men with symptomatic vertebral fractures commonly complain of back pain, loss of height and kyphosis, but they also have significantly less energy, poor sleep, more emotional problems and impaired mobility compared with age-matched control individuals (Scane et al. 1999).

Management (Figure 3.2)

In the past traditional management of acute vertebral fractures concentrated on analgesia, rest with some form of additional physical support followed by subsequent gradual immobilization within the

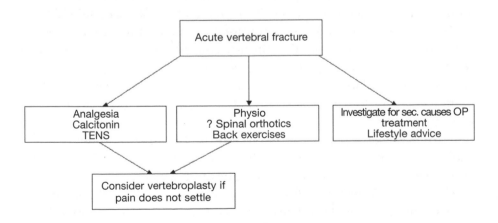

Figure 3.2 Management of acute vertebral fracture. TENS, transcutaneous electrical nerve stimulation.

limits of pain. Initially, strong opiates may be required but it is important to maintain a balance between pain relief while avoiding the
potential adverse effects of strong analgesics. Non-steroidal anti-
inflammatory drugs may also be helpful if they can be tolerated.
Transcutaneous electrical nerve stimulation (TENS) may prove valu-
able in the short term and intercostal nerve blocks may be helpful if
other measures prove ineffective. Specific bone active drugs may also
be used in the acute management of vertebral fractures. Both intramuscular and intranasal calcitonin have been shown to be strongly
analgesic within 2 weeks and this beneficial effect has persisted for at
least 4 months without serious side effects.

In addition to the use of analgesia physical measures may decrease
pain and facilitate mobilization. The mechanism by which exercise
decreases pain is not totally understood but improving axial muscle
strength by strengthening the back extensors has been shown to
decrease pain, and to reduce both spinal bone loss and the incidence
of further fractures (Sinaki et al. 2002). Long-term follow-up of women
who performed back extensor exercises for at least 2 years after a fracture have suggested that strength persists with possible reduction in
height loss (Sinaki et al. 2002).

The use of spinal orthotics in the acute phase may help to support
the spine, consequently reducing motion and reducing pain.
However, to avoid atrophy of supported back muscles, the use of
spinal supports needs to be discontinued as soon as pain subsides. At
the chronic back pain stage, a number of small studies have shown
that posture training spinal orthotics can be used to decrease pain
related to kyphotic deformity and secondary pain caused by over-
stretched ligamentous structures of the spine (Kaplan et al. 1996).
Pfeifer et al. (2004) demonstrated that wearing an orthosis for a 6-
month period increased trunk muscle strength, thus improving
posture in patients with vertebral fractures. An improved quality of life
was achieved by pain reduction, decrease in limitations of daily living
and improvement in well-being (Pfeifer et al. 2004).

The National Institute for Health and Clinical Excellence (NICE
2003a) published final guidance for vertebroplasty in September 2003.
This is an interventional radiological technique that involves the injection of bone cement, usually polymethylmethacrylate, into a cervical,
thoracic or lumbar vertebra. It is extremely effective for the relief of
pain from fracture that has not responded to conventional treatments

and appears to provide permanent pain relief in 80–90% of appropriately selected patients (Kallmes and Jensen 2003). Almost all the significant complications of vertebroplasty relate to cement leakage and, although rare, these can include spinal cord injury and exiting root injury with intravascular leakage that results in pulmonary embolus.

The technique of kyphoplasty is a frequently performed procedure in the USA. This involves the inflation of a balloon within the fractured vertebra to reduce kyphosis and form a cavity, subsequently filled with bone cement. It is likely that this procedure will have to be performed at multiple levels in an individual patient to produce a useful reduction in kyphosis, whereas pain relief is unlikely to be much different to that achieved by vertebroplasty. In November 2003, NICE (2003b) issued guidance on kyphoplasty, stating that there is, as yet, insufficient long-term evidence about the risks and benefits of the procedure and that it should be performed only in selected cases with special arrangements for patient consent.

Both vertebroplasty and kyphoplasty are intended to relieve pain in patients who have not responded to conservative measures and time. There is no clear evidence as to how long to wait before treating with vertebroplasty, but consensus is currently that a minimum of 4 weeks should pass and many practitioners will wait 6–8 weeks.

Hip fractures

Hip fracture represents the most serious complication of osteoporosis accounting for nearly 10% of all fractures with a much higher proportion in elderly people. It is associated with an estimated 10–12% probability of death during the first year after fracture and approximately half the survivors will suffer from long-term disability.

Epidemiology

It has been estimated that about 1.7 million hip fractures occurred world wide in 1990 (Cooper et al. 1992). The incidence of hip fracture increases exponentially with age in both men and women but, at all ages beyond 50 years, the incidence in women is about twice that in men. Although there has been the suggestion that hip fracture incidence may have levelled off in North America and Europe, it is rising rapidly in developing Asian countries (Lau 2001). With an expected increase in the world population and an increase in life expectancy, it has been estimated that globally the number of hip fractures could rise to 6.25 million by 2050 (Cooper et al. 1992).

Incidence rates in hip fractures vary substantially from one population to another with hip fracture being far more common among whites, than among non-whites. There is also substantial variation within populations of a given race and gender, with the incidence in North America and Europe varying more than sevenfold from one country to another (Johnell et al. 1992), thus suggesting an important role for environmental factors.

Within the UK hip fractures account for up to 9% of all limb fractures, with the lifetime risk from age 50 years being 14% in women and 3% in men. In 1997 Johansen and colleagues estimated that 2.28 hip fractures occurred annually per 1000 of the female population, with the corresponding figure for males being 0.61 per 1000. Extrapolated to the UK population of 59 million, it is expected that there will be 68 640 female hip fractures and 17 768 male hip fractures per year (Torgerson 2000). The cost of hip fracture comprises several components, including patient costs, post-fracture outpatient and GP care, and long-term institutional care. The annual cost of one hip fracture was estimated to be about £12 000 in 1998 (Dolan and Torgerson 1998). This estimate, however, covered only the first year of costs and, when these are updated to include nursing home and residential costs for a second year, the figure is likely to be £13 000 for the first year and £7000 for the subsequent year after fracture (Torgerson 2000).

Risk factors

Several factors contribute to the development of hip fracture including BMD, bone architecture, previous fracture history and other factors associated with physical frailty, and an increased risk of falls.

In patients with hip fracture, BMD is low in the hip, radius, lumbar spine and calcaneus, with low BMD at the hip site being the strongest predictor of future fracture. In women aged 65 and older, those with BMD in the lowest quartile have been shown to have an 8.5-fold greater risk of hip fracture than those in the highest quartile (Cummings et al. 1995). BMD measurements are known to predict fracture risk in the short term and femoral neck BMD appears to predict subsequent fractures up to 20 years later (Melton et al. 2003). After hip fracture BMD may continue to decrease at the non-fractured hip by 4–5% in the first year, subsequently increasing the risk of further fracture (Dirschl et al. 2000).

The geometric characteristics of bone have been implicated in the risk of hip fracture in women, with the risk being significantly higher in white women who have a longer hip axis length than Asian or black women (Cummings et al. 1995).

In both men and women the risk of hip fracture is increased by a previous fracture at any site. In those who have already suffered a hip fracture, the odds ratio of a second fracture is increased six- to eightfold (Chaapurlat et al. 2003). Men and women aged 65 years or older with a vertebral fracture have a 5-year rate of a risk of hip fracture of 6.7% and 13.3%, respectively (Van Staa et al. 2002); in addition the relative risk of hip fracture increases after wrist fractures in both sexes.

The identification of clinical predictors has not been easy and generally clinical risk factors are poor at predicting low BMD or fractures with only 17–27% of postmenopausal women at risk of hip fractures being readily identified in this way. The relevant clinical risk factors that may be important include a maternal history of hip fracture, treatment with long-acting benzodiazepines or anticonvulsant drugs, ingestion of excess caffeine, spending 4 hours a day or less on their feet and a history of current smoking. Women with a reduced BMI and those who reported their health as poor were also at increased risk. Examination factors associated with increased risk include the inability to rise from a chair without using one's arms, poor depth perception, poor contrast sensitivity and tachycardia at rest (Cummings et al. 1995).

Consequences

Hip fractures are associated with considerable trauma in elderly patients, who typically have other serious underlying diseases. In the acute phase, most evidence guiding perioperative risk management of patients undergoing surgery focuses on cardiac and thromboembolic risk. A large study of 8930 patients reported in 2002 (Lawrence et al. 2002) showed that 19% of patients had a postoperative medical condition with cardiac and pulmonary complications being the most common. The 30-day mortality was similar for serious cardiac and pulmonary complications and patients with multiple complications had a particularly poor prognosis.

More important in some respects than acute medical complications is the devastating loss of function that frequently follows a hip fracture. Past and recent studies have demonstrated that about 40% of patients are unable to walk independently 1 year after hip fracture (Cooper 1997, Lin and Chang 2004), and 60% have limitations in at least one class 1 activity of daily living (e.g. feeding, dressing, toileting) and 80% are limited in a class 2 activity (e.g. shopping, gardening, housework). Although there are age-related declines in function with respect to the activities of daily living, it has been shown that hip fracture patients have substantially more disability than could be explained by ageing over 24 months (Magaziner et al. 2003) (Figures 3.3 and 3.4). In the first year after hip fracture approximately 27% of patients will require nursing home care and 30% will require additional home support. Of the patients who were independent before a hip fracture, 18% become dependent and 8% require nursing home care (Cooper 1997).

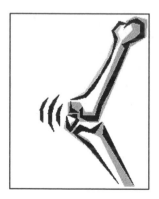

59% deteriorated functionally

29% confined to bed or chair

60% used walking aid

13% required analgesia for pain

Figure 3.3 Lifestyle change after hip fracture.

Hip fractures are also associated with increased mortality with most deaths occurring in the first days and months after the fracture. Kanis and colleagues (2003) have suggested that approximately a quarter of

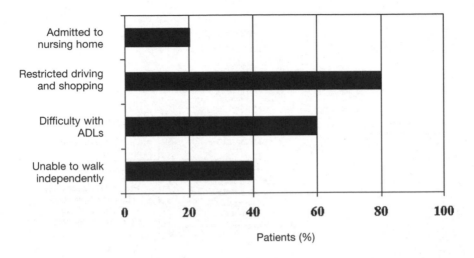

Figure 3.4 Morbidity after hip fractures. ADLs, activities of daily living. (From Cooper 1997.)

early deaths are related to the fracture itself but other studies have shown that a smaller minority could be attributed to the fracture itself. Life expectancy is reduced by hip fracture with this mortality being greater in men than women at all ages over 50 years. This excess mortality is however restricted to patients with reduced mental status, reduced general health and low physical ability (Poor et al. 1995).

Management (Figure 3.5)

The National Confidential Enquiry into Perioperative Deaths 1999, entitled *Extremes of Age*, stated that: 'A team of senior surgeons, anaesthetists and physicians needs to be closely involved in the care of elderly patients who have poor physical status and high operative risk' (Callum et al. 1999, p. 551) – a description that is all too apt for too many elderly patients with hip fractures. Time spent in the accident and emergency department should be minimal and many clinicians advocate a fast-track system for hip fracture patients, with rapid assessment and symptom relief. However, the current pressure on departments nationally to move all patients through in 4 hours makes this goal difficult to attain. Before surgery it is essential that the patient undergoes a full clinical evaluation with assessment of mental state, hydration, cardiac rhythm and cardiorespiratory status. Medication

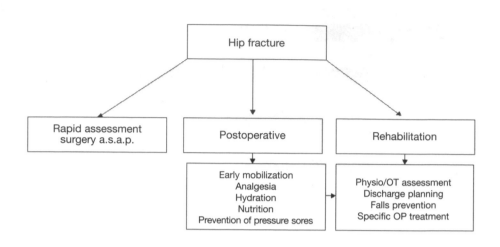

Figure 3.5 Management of hip fracture. OP, osteoporosis; OT, occupational therapist.

should be assessed on admission and appropriate changes considered before surgery when relevant. Routine investigations should include hip and chest radiographs, haematological and biochemical profiles, and an electrocardiogram.

A full social history, including information on type of dwelling, activities of daily living and the family and other support systems, is also relevant.

For optimum pain control, early mobilization and functional recovery surgery should occur within 24 hours if the patient is medically fit and should be performed by experienced surgeons and anaesthetists. The type of surgery required remains slightly controversial but, over the past few years, several randomized controlled trials have indicated the superiority of arthroplasty instead of internal fixation for femoral neck fractures, particularly when the fracture is severely displaced (Obrant 2004). Many of the problems encountered in the peri- and postoperative periods are indicative of the impaired physiological reserve capacity that comes with advancing years, particularly in those with associated co-morbidity. Common complications include urinary tract infection, pressure sores, chest infection, thromboembolism and sepsis. Delirium is not uncommon and can be the result of a variety of avoidable problems, including pain, use of opiate-containing analgesics, infection, hypoxaemia, and fluid and electrolyte imbalance.

Postoperative care should focus on the priorities of early mobilization and the prevention of medical complications with daily assessments of cardiorespiratory status, fluid balance, analgesia, thromboprophylaxis, pressure sore prevention and adequate nutrition. Hip fracture patients are highly catabolic and often present in a suboptimal nutritional state and therefore supplementation of a hospital diet may be necessary. There is some evidence to show improved functional outcomes and impact on length of stay when nutritional intake is actively monitored and the diet supplemented with high protein foods (Avenell and Handholl 2004).

After surgery most hip fracture patients will benefit from a period of rehabilitation, ideally in a specialized unit with early involvement of a multidisciplinary team including medical and nursing staff, occupational therapists, physiotherapists and social workers. There is no one model of care that has been shown to be significantly better than the others but data support the use of orthogeriatric units in terms of improving likelihood of returning to original place of residence (Cameron et al. 2000). Patients with a good prefracture level of mobility and lack of cognitive impairment tend to benefit most from rehabilitation schemes (Aitken and Yu 1998). The period in rehabilitation depends on the individual and the availability of resources, but may be in excess of 30 days.

In an attempt to reduce further fractures, all patients who have sustained a hip fracture should be offered advice on lifestyle measures to decrease bone loss, including eating a balanced diet rich in calcium, minimizing tobacco and alcohol consumption, and maintaining regular exercise and adequate exposure to sunlight. In the group of frail elderly patients who have sustained a hip fracture it is probably inappropriate to perform substantial investigations to exclude secondary causes of osteoporosis or to confirm the diagnosis of osteoporosis by bone densitometry. These patients are more likely to benefit from calcium and vitamin D supplementation than from other therapeutic interventions (Chapuy et al. 1992). Those patients who are slightly younger and more mobile before fracture may also benefit from calcium and vitamin D, more active investigation and possible treatment with a bisphosphonate.

Once discharged from hospital it is important that the rehabilitation process continues in the home environment with emphasis on independence where possible. Patients should be given the opportunity to progress mobility further and outdoor mobility should be considered as a goal for those previously able to go out alone.

Hip protectors

As the majority of hip fractures are caused by a fall with direct impact on the greater trochanter, an option for fracture prevention would be to divert this impact. A specially designed external hip protector positioned over the trochanteric region serves to weaken the impacting force and energy of the fall, diverting from the greater trochanter into the surrounding soft tissues. Early work by Lauritzen and colleagues (1993) demonstrated a 50% reduction in hip fracture incidence in residents of elderly care homes. A further randomized controlled trial in 2000 (Kannus et al. 2000) showed, with an intention-to-treat analysis, that the risk of hip fracture was 60% less in the group who wore hip protectors. Since publication of the first trials evaluating the effects of hip protectors, there has been a rapid increase in the variety of devices available on the market. Many types of these devices are available with unsubstantiated claims for fracture prevention and very few models have been studied systematically or scientifically (Kannus et al. 2003). The newest models emphasize a thin design in an attempt to increase comfort and compliance, but this is most probably achieved at the expense of reduced force attenuation, efficacy and safety.

The initial promise shown by hip protectors does not appear to have been sustained, with unresolved controversies over ideal type, fit, quality control and patient compliance. Parker and colleagues (2003), on reviewing seven randomized controlled trials involving more than 3000 patients, were unable to demonstrate any significant benefit to those wearing hip protectors. The study of Birks et al. (2004) in 4169 women, aged 70 years or more with a risk for hip fracture, showed no significant reduction in hip fracture incidence in those wearing hip protectors, with only 31% of study participants continuing to wear them on a daily basis.

Wrist fractures

A Colles' fracture that is usually explained by a fall onto an outstretched arm is one of the most common sites of osteoporotic fracture and contributes to significant morbidity. More than 40 000 Colles' fractures occur each year in the UK, accounting for about 23% of all limb fractures sustained. They are more common in women with a steep rise in incidence between the ages of 40 and 65 years, followed by a plateau thereafter. In men there is no apparent increase in incidence of wrist fracture with age, with it remaining relatively constant between 20 and 80 years (Cooper and Melton 1992). The incidence of wrist fractures varies with geographical location and time of the year, with greater numbers during winter, probably related to falls outside on an icy surface. Although this fracture accrues costs associated with outpatient visits and loss of working days, in the younger person it does not usually necessitate long-term hospitalization and it is estimated that annual costs of each fracture are about £468.

Risk factors

As with other osteoporotic fractures there is an association between low BMD and fracture risk. Predictions of the incidence of Colles' fracture in the general population, based on BMD alone, are very close to the observed incidence, suggesting that low BMD is a major determinant of Colles' fracture. In the SOF, women in the lowest quintile of BMD measurements had four times the risk of fracture compared with those in the highest quintile (Kelsey et al. 1992). In the Dubbo study (Nguyen et al. 2001), increased fracture risk was associated with low femoral neck bone density in both sexes. A Colles' fracture is also a useful indicator of an increased risk of hip fracture in older people and one series of 1288 men and women with forearm fracture showed a fivefold increase in risk among women and a tenfold increase in men in the risk of vertebral fracture.

Few lifestyle factors have been shown to be predictive of future Colles' fracture in either sex. Several studies have suggested only a limited role for physical inactivity, smoking, body mass and co-morbidity (Silman 2002). Low dietary calcium intake in men and a history of falls and delayed menarche in women are potentially related to increased risk of fracture. Regular activity in advancing age may confer a greater risk, reflecting the increased exposure to risk of falling (Silman 2002). As wrist fractures tend to be related to falls, the general characteristics that predict falling, including poor eyesight, postural instability and general frailty, are also relevant in the prediction of wrist fractures.

Consequences

Although fractures of the wrist cause less morbidity than those of the hip – they are very rarely fatal and seldom require hospitalization – the consequences are often underestimated. The need for hospitalization rises with age and 70% of patients aged 85 years or over may require hospital care for a short time. Prospective studies show that there is a high incidence of algodystrophy after Colles' fracture, which causes pain, stiffness, swelling and vasomotor disturbances of the hand. Although the disorder commonly resolves spontaneously after a year, many patients will have residual stiffness. Other complications include malunion, resulting in deformity and swelling. Several studies suggest that mortality is not higher among women with Colles' fracture than among the general population (Kanis 1994).

Management

Colles' fracture alone is not sufficiently predictive of risk of osteo-porosis to warrant therapeutic intervention, without further assessment of BMD and consideration of additional risk factors. In patients aged 65–75 with a low-impact Colles' fracture osteoporosis should be considered and BMD measured by dual energy X-ray absorptiometry (DXA) where possible. Those with a T score (bone density value commonly expressed in standard deviation units with reference to the young normal range consisting of individuals at peak bone mass) below –2.5 SD warrant investigation for any secondary causes of osteoporosis and should be treated accordingly. All patients should be offered lifestyle advice on diet, exercise and fall prevention if appropriate. Treatment with a bisphosphonate should be considered with additional calcium and vitamin D supplementation in frail elderly people.

Falls and fractures

Compromised bone strength and falling, alone, or more frequently in combination, are the two main independent and immediate risk factors for fractures in elderly people. In the community, 30% of people over the age of 65 years fall each year and more than half of those living in long-term care fall every year, some repeatedly (Tinetti and

Speechley 1989). Recurrent falls are associated with increased mortality, increased rate of hospitalization, curtailment of daily activities, increased fear of falling, loss of confidence, and higher rates of institutionalization and mortality (Campbell et al. 1990, Tinetti and Williams 1997). Between 10 and 25% of falls result in serious injury and up to 6% culminate in a fracture (Campbell et al. 1990). More than 95% of hip fractures occur in association with a fall, and the highest risk of fracture is observed in those who have osteoporosis and are also at the highest risk of falling (Grisso et al. 1991).

When a person falls, the type and severity of the fall, characterized by height and energy, fall direction, mechanics and anatomical site of the impact, are crucial in determining whether or not a fracture occurs. In attempting to explain the implied underlying causal processes involved, numerous studies have identified over 400 potential risk factors for falling, the most important of which include those related to the environment, gait/balance disorders or weakness, dizziness and vertigo, use of assistive devices, impaired activities of daily living, chronic diseases and polypharmacy (Rubenstein and Josephson 2002).

Randomized controlled trials of falls prevention strategies have focused on both multifactorial and unifactorial approaches. It is likely that the multifactorial approach will yield more benefits but this approach has limitations, because it may be difficult to distinguish between the independent role of each modified risk factor, therefore making it impossible to determine which part of the intervention is effective and which is not. However, the Yale multifactorial study 'Frailty and Injuries: Co-operative Studies of Intervention Techniques', which included review of medications, balance and gait training and improvement of functional skills, showed a significant 31% reduction in falls at 1 year (Tinetti et al. 1994). The 'Prevention of Falls in the Elderly Trial' in the UK showed that a structured multifactorial medical and occupational therapy assessment in the follow-up of older people presenting to the accident and emergency department with a fall produced a significant reduction in the number of recurrent falls (Close et al. 1999). Multifactorial intervention in those with impaired cognition attending A&E after a fall failed to show a positive effect (Shaw et al. 2003). This observation of the poor response of older people with a low level of cognition has also been confirmed among elderly people living in residential care settings

(Jensen et al. 2003). Unifactorial interventions, which include individually targeted exercise programmes emphasizing strength and balance, have been shown to redsuce the incidence of falls and injuries significantly (Carter et al. 2001, Robertson et al. 2001). Psychotrophic medication withdrawal can significantly reduce the risk of falling but permanent withdrawal is difficult to achieve (Campbell et al. 1999). The benefits of unifactorial home assessments by occupational therapists are currently controversial. It has been shown that home visits can prevent falls but much of the fall reduction occurred outside the home, suggesting that behaviour modification, rather than environmental modification, may be the reason for the beneficial effect (Cumming et al. 1999).

A recent clinical guideline produced by the NICE (2004) has commented on the use of multifactorial falls risk assessment emphasizing the importance of strength and balance training, home hazard assessment and intervention, vision assessment and referral and medication review and cardiac pacing where appropriate (Figure 3.6). Although the evidence is not so strong it also recommends that the older person at risk of falls should be encouraged to participate in falls prevention programmes including education and information giving. Options not recommended included low intensity or untargeted group exercises and unifactorial cognitive–behavioural interventions.

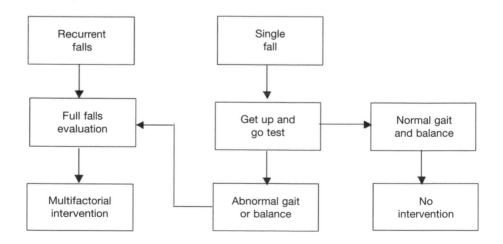

Figure 3.6 Falls assessment and management.

Multifactorial falls risk assessment

- Falls history
- Gait, balance and mobility, muscle weakness
- Osteoporosis risk
- Perceived functional ability and fear of falling
- Visual impairment
- Cognitive impairment
- Urinary incontinence
- Home hazards
- Cardiovascular examination
- Medication review

NICE (2004)

Multifactorial interventions

- Strength and balance training
- Home hazard assessment and intervention
- Vision assessment and referral
- Medication review with modification
- Identify future risk
- Participation in falls prevention programmes with written and verbal information

NICE (2004)

The high rate of osteoporotic fracture in western populations has resulted in a significant burden in terms of morbidity, mortality, and health and social care costs. As the health of large populations improves and life expectancy increases, fracture incidence will also increase. There are many intrinsic and extrinsic risk factors for fractures that have been proven at an epidemiological level; early recognition of these may help to prevent both initial and subsequent fractures. Early acute management of fractures with continuing rehabilitation where necessary should aim to improve outcomes and maximize quality of life.

References

Aitken E, Yu G (1998) Orthogeriatric rehabilitation: Which patients benefit most? Hosp Med 59(4): 274–6.

Avenell A, Handholl HH (2004) Nutritional supplementation for hip fracture after care in the elderly. Cochrane Database Systematic Review (1). CD001880.

Begerow B, Pfeifer M, Pospeschill M et al. (1999) Time since vertebral fracture: An important variable concerning quality of life in patients with postmenopausal osteoporosis. Osteopor Int 10: 26–33.

Birks Y, Porthouse J, Addie C et al. (2004) Randomised controlled trial of hip protectors among women living in the community. Osteopor Int 15: 701–6.

Black D, Arden NK, Paalermo L, Peaarsson J, Cummings SR (1999) Prevalent vertebral deformities predict hip fractures and new vertebral deformities but not wrist fractures. J Bone Miner Res 14: 821–8.

Burge RT, Worley D, Johansen A et al. (2001) The cost of osteoporotic fractures in the UK: Projections for 2000–2020. J Med Econ 4: 51–62.

Callum KG, Gray AJG, Hoile RW et al. (1999) Extremes of Age. National Confidential Enquiry into Perioperative Deaths. National Confidential Enquiry into Patient Outcome and Death (NCEPOD), p. 55.

Cameron ID, Handholl HH, Finnegan TP, Madhok R, Langhorne P (2000) Co-ordinated multi-disciplinary approaches for in patient rehabilitation of older patients with proximal femoral fracture. Cochrane Database System (4). CD000106 Review.

Campbell AJ, Borrie MJ, Spears GF, Jackson SL, Brown JS, Fitzgerald JL (1990) Circumstances and consequences of falls experienced by a community population 70 years and over during a prospective study. Age Ageing 19: 136–41.

Campbell AJ, Robertson MC, Gardner MM, Norton RN, Buchner DM (1999) Psychotropic medication withdrawal and a home based exercise programme to prevent falls: A randomised controlled trial. J Am Geriatr Soc 47: 850–3.

Caplan G, Scane AC, Francis RM (1994) Pathogenesis of vertebral crush fracture in women. J R Soc Med 87: 200–2.

Carter N, Kannus P, Khan KM (2001) Exercise in the prevention of falls in older people: A systematic literature review examining the rationale and the evidence. Sports Med 31: 427–38.

Chaapurlat RD, Bauer DC, Nevitt M, Stone K, Cummings SR (2003) Incidence and risk factors for a second hip fracture in elderly women. The Study of Osteoporotic Fractures. Osteopor Int 14: 130–6.

Chapuy MC, Arlot ME, Duboeuf F et al. (1992). Vitamin D and calcium to prevent hip fractures in elderly women. N Engl J Med 327: 1637–42.

Close J, Ellis M, Hooper R, Glucksman E, Jackson S, Swift C (1999) Prevention of Falls in the Elderly Trial (PROFET): A randomised controlled trial. Lancet 353: 93–7.

Cooper C (1993) Epidemiology and public health impact of osteoporosis. In: Reid DM (ed.), Clinical Rheumatology: Osteoporosis. London: Baillière Tindall, PP. 459–77.

Cooper C (1997) The crippling consequences of fractures and their impact on quality of life. Am J Med 103(suppl 2a): 12–19s.

Cooper C, Melton LJ III (1992) Epidemiology of osteoporosis. TEM 3: 224–9.

Cooper C, Campion G, Melton LJ III (1992) Hip fracture in the elderly. A worldwide projection. Osteopor Int 2: 285–9.

Cumming RG, Thomas M, Szonyi G et al. (1999) Home visits by an occupational therapist for assessment and modification of environmental hazards: A randomised trial of falls prevention. J Am Geriatr Soc 47: 1471–81.

Cummings SR, Nevitt MC, Browner WS et al. (1995) The Study of Osteoporotic Fractures Research Group. Risk factors for hip fracture in white women. N Engl J Med 332: 767–73.

Delmas PD, Eastell R, Gaarnero P et al. (2000). The use of biochemical markers of bone turnover in osteoporosis. Osteopor Int 11(suppl 6): 2–17.

Dennison E, Cooper C (1996) The epidemiology of osteoporosis. Br J Clin Pract 50: 33–6.

Dirschl DR, Piedrahita L, Henderson RC (2000) Bone mineral density 6 years after a hip fracture: A prospective, longitudinal study. Bone 26: 95–8.

Dolan P, Torgerson DJ (1998) The costs of treating osteoporotic fractures in the United Kingdom female population. Osteopor Int 8: 611–17.

Eastell R, Reid DM, Compston J et al. (2001) Secondary prevention of osteoporosis. When should a non vertebral fracture be a trigger for action? Q J Med 94: 575–97.

Faulkner KG, Cummings SR, Nevitt MC, Pressman A, Jergas M, Genant HC (1995) Study of osteoporotic fracture research group. Hip axis length and osteoporotic fracture. J Bone Miner Res 10: 506–8.

Grisso JA, Kelsey JL, Strom BL et al. (1991) Risk factors for falls as a cause of hip fracture in women. The Northeast Hip Fracture Study Group. N Engl J Med 324: 1326–31.

Hall SE, Criddle RA, Comito TL, Prince RL (1999) A case control study of quality of life and functional impairment in women with long standing vertebral osteoporotic fractures. Osteopor Int 9: 508–15.

Jensen J, Nyberg L, Gustafson Y, Lundin-Olsson L (2003) Fall and injury prevention in residential care-effects in residents with higher and lower levels of cognition. J Am Geriatr Soc 51: 627–35.

Johansen A, Evans RJ, Stone MD, Richmond PW et al. (1997). Fracture incidence in England and Wales: A study based on the population of Cardiff. Injury 28: 655–60.

Johnell O, Gullberg B, Allander E, Kanis JA (1992) The apparent incidence of hip fracture in Europe: A study of national register sources. MEDOS Study Group. Osteopor Int 2: 298–302.

Kado DM, Browner WS, Palermo L, Nevitt MC, Genant HK, Cummings SR (1999) Vertebral fractures and mortality in older women: A prospective study. Study of Osteoporotic Fractures Research Group. Arch Intern Med 159: 1215–20.

Kallmes DF, Jensen ME (2003) Percutaneous vertebroplasty. Radiology 229: 27–36.

Kanis JA (1994) Osteoporosis. Oxford: Blackwell Science Ltd.

Kanis JA, Oden A, Johnell O, De Laet C, Jonsson B, Oglesby AK (2003) The components of excess mortality after hip fracture. Bone 32: 468–73.

Kannus P, Parkkari J, Niemi S et al. (2000) Prevention of hip fractures in elderly people with use of a hip protector. N Engl J Med 343: 1506–13.

Kannus P, Parkkari J, Khan K (2003) Hip protectors need an evidence base. Lancet 362: 1168–9.

Kaplan RS, Sinaki M, Hameister MD (1996) Effect of back supports on back strength in patients with osteoporosis: A pilot study. Mayo Clin Proc 71: 235–41.

Kelsey JL, Browner WS, Seeley DG, Nevitt MC, Cummings SR (1992) Risk factors for fractures of the distal forearm and proximal humerus. The Study of Osteoporotic Fractures Research Group. Am J Epidemiol 135: 477–89.

Lau EM (2001) Epidemiology of osteoporosis. In: Woolf AD (ed), Best Practice and Research: Clinical Rheumatology 15(3). London: Bailliere Tindal.

Lauritzen JB, Petersen MM, Lund B (1993) Effect of external hip protectors on hip fractures. Lancet 341: 11–13.

Lawrence VA, Hilsenbeck SG, Noveck H, Poses RM, Carson JL (2002) Medical complications and outcomes after hip fracture repair. Arch Intern Med 162: 2053–7.

Lin PC, Chang SY (2004) Functional recovery among elderly people one year after hip surgery. J Nurs Res 12(1): 72–82.

Magaziner J, Fredman L, Hawkes W et al. (2003) Changes in functional status attributable to hip fracture patients to community dwelling aged. Am J Epidemiol 157: 1023–31.

Melton LG, Crowson CS, O'Fallon WM, Wahner HW, Riggs BL (2003) Relative contributions of bone density, bone turnover, and clinical risk factors to long term fracture prediction. J Bone Miner Res 18: 312–18.

National Institute for Clinical Excellence (2003a) Percutaneous Vertebroplasty. London: NICE.

National Institute for Clinical Excellence (2003b) Balloon Kyphoplasty for Vertebral Compression Fractures. London: NICE.

National Institute for Clinical Excellence (2004) Falls: The assessment and prevention of falls in older people. London: NICE.

Nguyen TV, Center JR, Sambrook PN, Eisman JA (2001) Risk factors for proximal humerus, forearm and wrist fracture in elderly men and women: The Dubbo Osteoporosis Epidemiology Study. Am J Epidemiol 153: 587–95.

O'Neill TW, Felsenberg B, Varlow J, Cooper C, Kanos JA, Silman AJ (1996) The prevalence of vertebral deformity in European men and women. The European Vertebral Osteoporosis Study. J Bone Miner Res 11: 1010–18.

O'Neill TW, Cockerill W, Matthis C et al. (2004) Back pain, disability and radiographic vertebral fracture in European women: A prospective study. Osteopor Int 15: 760–5.

Obrant K (2004) Fracture management in osteoporosis. In: Woolf AD, Akesson K, Adami S (eds), The Year in Osteoporosis, Vol. 1. Clinical Publishing. Oxford: Atlas Medical Publishing, pp. 283–93.

Parker MJ, Gillespie LD, Gillespie WJ (2003) Hip protectors for preventing hip fractures in the elderly. Cochrane Review. Cochrane Library: Issue 1.

Pfeifer M, Begerow B, Minne HW (2004) Effects of a new spinal orthosis on posture, trunk strength, and quality of life in women with postmenopausal osteoporosis: a randomized trial. Am J Phys Med Rehabil 83: 177–86.

Poor G, Atkinson EJ, O'Fallon WM, Melton LJ III (1995) Determinants of reduced survival following hip fractures in men. Clin Orthop 319: 260–5.

Robertson MC, Devlin N, Gardner MM, Campbell AY (2001) Effectiveness and economic evaluation of a nurse delivered home exercise programme to prevent falls. BMJ 322: 697–701.

Roy DK, O'Neill TW, Finn JD (2003) Determinants of incident vertebral fracture in men and women: Results for the European Prospective Osteoporosis Study (EPOS). Osteopor Int 14: 19–26

Rubenstein LZ, Josephson KR (2002) The epidemiology of falls and syncope. Clin Geriatr Med 18: 141–58.

Scane AC, Francis RM, Sutcliffe AM (1999) Case control study of the pathogenesis and sequelae of symptomatic vertebral fractures in men. Osteopor Int 9: 91–7.

Shaw FE, Bond J, Richardson DA et al. (2003) Multifactorial intervention after a fall in older people with cognitive impairment and dementia presenting to the accident and emergency department: Randomised controlled trial. BMJ 326: 73–8.

Silman AJ (2002) Risk factors for Colles' fracture in men and women: Results from the European Prospective Osteoporosis Study. Osteopor Int 14: 213–18.

Silman AJ, O'Neill TW, Cooper C, Kanis J, Felsenberg D (1997) Influence of physical activity on vertebral deformity in men and women: Results from the European Vertebral Osteoporosis Study. J Bone Miner Res 12: 813–19.

Sinaki M, Itoi E, Wahner HW et al. (2002) Stronger back muscles reduce the incidence of vertebral fractures: A prospective 10 year follow up of postmenopausal women. Bone 30: 836–41.

Tinetti ME, Speechley M (1989) Prevention of falls among the elderly. N Engl J Med 320: 1055–9.

Tinetti ME, Williams CS (1997) Falls, injuries due to falls, and the risk of admission to a nursing home. N Engl J Med 337: 1279–84.

Tinetti ME, Baker DI, McAvay G et al. (1994) A multifactorial intervention to reduce the risk of falling among elderly people living in the community. N Engl J Med 331: 821–7.

Torgerson DJ (2000) The cost of treating osteoporotic fractures in the United Kingdom female population. Osteopor Int 11: 551–2.

Van der Klift M, De Laet CE, McCloskey EV, Hofman A, Pols HA (2002) The incidence of vertebral fractures in men and women: The Rotterdam Study. J Bone Miner Res: 17: 1051–6.

Van Staa TP, Leufkens HGM, Cooper C (2002) Does a fracture at one site predict later fracture at other sites? A British cohort study. Osteopor Int 13: 624–9.

World Health Organization (1994) Assessment of Fracture Risk and Its Application to Screening for Postmenopausal Osteoporosis. Technical Report Series 843. Geneva: WHO.

CHAPTER 4

Lifestyle factors and osteoporosis

- Nutritional factors are important to maintain skeletal integrity
- Tobacco consumption may adversely affect bone density
- The most compelling evidence for a beneficial effect of exercise on bone density is during childhood and adolescence with current and past exercise preventing hip fracture

The effect of lifestyle measures on the attainment of peak bone mass and prevention of bone loss and fractures has been well documented. This chapter discusses the influence of diet, particularly calcium intake and the role of vitamin D, with passing reference to the potential benefits of fruit and vegetables. The second part of the chapter examines the effects of exercise on the skeleton from childhood through to advanced age.

Dietary intake (Figure 4.1)

The influence of nutrient intake on bone mineral density (BMD) is still largely undefined but nutritional factors are clearly of importance to bone health, because they may be modifiable. Evidence suggests that calcium intake is important during skeletal growth and peak bone mass development, and there is a general consensus of agreement that calcium may be effective in reducing bone loss in late postmenopausal women, particularly in those with habitual low dietary calcium intake. Vitamin D is also necessary for optimal absorption of calcium and there are some promising data showing a positive impact of vitamin D on reducing postmenopausal bone loss. Recent evidence now suggests a link between fruit and vegetable intake and bone health, and the emergence of biologically active compounds found in various

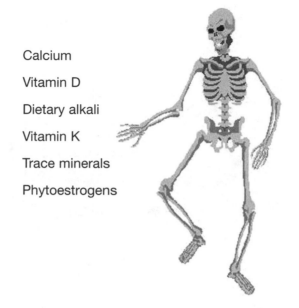

Calcium

Vitamin D

Dietary alkali

Vitamin K

Trace minerals

Phytoestrogens

Figure 4.1 Diet and prevention of osteoporosis.

foodstuffs known as phytoestrogens has also prompted research on the effects on bone density.

Calcium and vitamin D metabolism

Calcium is required for a number of functions in the body including neuromuscular activity, membrane function, hormone secretion, enzyme activity, coagulation of the blood and skeletal mineralization (Francis 1996). Over 99% of the body's calcium is stored in bone, where it provides mechanical strength to the skeleton and serves as a mineral reservoir, which can be drawn upon to maintain a normal plasma calcium. Calcium is absorbed from the small bowel by an active transport mechanism and by passive diffusion, this active transport being regulated by the circulating levels of 1,25-dihydroxyvitamin D ($1,25[OH]_2D$), the hormonally active metabolite of vitamin D (Figure 4.2).

Once absorbed, calcium enters the circulation, where it exchanges with the cellular and skeletal calcium. Plasma calcium concentration is

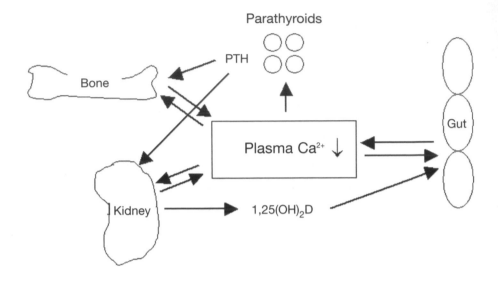

Figure 4.2 Calcium metabolism. 1,25(OH)$_2$D, 1,25-dihydroxyvitamin D; PTH, parathyroid hormone.

regulated by the actions of parathyroid hormone (PTH) and the vitamin D endocrine system on the bowel, kidneys and skeleton (Francis 1996). The major source of vitamin D is from the skin, following exposure to ultraviolet radiation. The diet provides much smaller amounts of vitamin D, but this source is essential when cutaneous production is limited because of lack of exposure to sunlight. Vitamin D has little biological activity and is metabolized in the liver to 25-hydroxyvitamin (25[OH]D), the major circulating metabolite of the vitamin; this then undergoes further hydroxylation in the kidneys to form 1,25(OH)$_2$D, which plays an important role, not only in the regulation of calcium absorption but also in bone mineralization and muscle function (Figure 4.3).

The body adapts to changes in dietary calcium intake by modifying calcium absorption and renal tubular reabsorption of calcium. If the dietary calcium intake is insufficient to offset the obligatory losses in the urine and faeces, calcium will be drained from the skeletal reservoir to maintain normal circulating levels. In childhood and adolescence, additional calcium is required for mineralization of the growing skeleton (Francis 1996). Individuals demonstrate great physiological adaptability in their

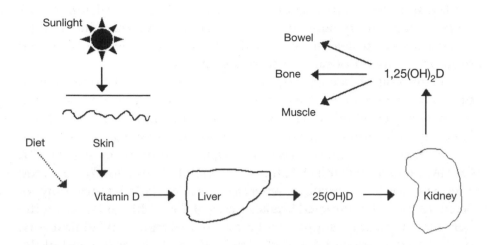

Figure 4.3 Vitamin D production and metabolism. 1,25(OH)$_2$D,
1,25-dihydroxyvitamin D; 25(OH)D, 25-hydroxyvitamin D.
(From Chapuy et al. 1992, 1994.)

absorption, excretion and metabolic use of dietary calcium, e.g. during periods of growth when the biological requirement is high,
calcium conservation mechanisms become more efficient if calcium
intake is low. There are also physiological changes in calcium and
bone metabolism during pregnancy and lactation to meet the
increased demand for calcium.

As bone is the major reservoir for calcium this has led to the view
that adequate calcium nutrition is important for the maintenance of
skeletal health. Professionals interested in osteoporosis, the National
Osteoporosis Society (NOS) and manufacturers of calcium supplements highlight the importance of dietary calcium intake in the
prevention and treatment of osteoporosis. In contrast, Plant and Tidey
(2003) have suggested that a high intake of calcium in dairy produce
may contribute to the development of osteoporosis, although the scientific basis of this view has been challenged (Francis and New 2003).
Many epidemiological studies show an association between the lifetime intake of calcium and either low bone density or a high risk of
fracture in women. In a recent comprehensive review of the literature,
Heaney (2002) examined the effects of calcium intake on the acquisition of bone during growth, on subsequent bone loss and on the
incidence of fractures later in life. The majority of 52 controlled

studies showed a beneficial effect of increased dietary calcium intake on bone acquisition, bone loss and fracture risk. Although most of the investigator-controlled studies used calcium supplements, those that used dairy sources of calcium were also positive.

The amount of calcium required for maximum peak bone mass in the younger person remains a topic of considerable debate, with differing opinions within and between different countries (Heaney 2000, Specker 2000). Some of these differences of opinion may be explained by the ways that countries have approached the problem, e.g. the UK COMA Committee (Table 4.1) has determined calcium intakes deemed adequate for a population whereas the US National Academy of Sciences panel has targeted intakes optimal for health. In assessing the benefits of calcium supplementation in children and adolescents, studies have suggested that BMD improves by 1–5% at the end of the intervention period. Earlier studies suggested that this increase in bone mass was more marked in prepubertal children; in addition earlier studies failed to show a difference in bone mass longitudinally, once the supplement was withdrawn. However, a number of recently published trials have suggested that the long-term benefits of supplementation on bone density are maintained, several years after discontinuation (Bonjour et al. 2001, Matkovic et al. 2003). It has also been suggested that greater gains in bone mass may be achieved when impact-loaded skeletal sites are subject to short bouts of moderate exercise combined with additional dietary calcium (Iuliano-Burns et al. 2003). In clinical and public health terms, advice to our younger population for improving their bone density must be centred on the requirement for both a physical activity regimen and a diet that is balanced and rich in dietary calcium.

Table 4.1 Calcium requirements: COMA recommendations

Age (years)	Daily intake (mg)
< 1	525
1–3	350
4–6	450
7–10	550
11–18	1000 (M)/800 (F)
19+	700

Bone loss begins between the ages of 35 and 40 in both sexes, but there is an accelerated rate of loss in the decade after the menopause in women. The role of dietary calcium intake and calcium supplementation in reducing peri- and postmenopausal bone loss remains controversial. Trials on the benefits of calcium supplementation in the early post-menopausal years (< 5 years) remain inconclusive. However, there is now a general consensus of opinion that calcium is effective in reducing bone loss in late (> 5 years) postmenopausal women, particularly in those with a low dietary calcium intake (< 400 mg/day). A meta-analysis of the relationship between calcium intake and fracture risk has suggested that a low dietary calcium intake predisposes to an increased risk of fracture (Cummings et al. 1995). In addition, a large case–control study of hip fracture risk in southern Europe demonstrated that exposure to a high dietary intake of calcium was associated with a significant decrease of the risk of hip fracture in both sexes (Johnell et al. 1995).

Older, frailer people who are either housebound or living in nursing homes are at greater risk of falling and fractures. It is now generally recognized that calcium and vitamin D are effective in reducing fracture rates in this population and supplementation should be considered as a matter of course. This treatment is generally safe and, although a few cases of hypercalcaemia have been reported, these are extremely rare. The major study of combined calcium and vitamin D supplementation in older people is that of Chapuy and colleagues, conducted in France in the early 1990s (Figure 4.4). This randomized controlled trial demonstrated a reduction of 23% in hip fractures and 17% reduction in non-vertebral fractures after 3 years of treatment in those women given supplementation (Chapuy et al. 1994). A recent Cochrane Review has compared the effects of combined calcium and vitamin D supplementation and vitamin D supplementation alone on the incidence of hip fractures (Gillespie et al. 2004). This showed a significant reduction in hip fractures in frail elderly people on combined calcium and vitamin D supplementation, but no decrease with vitamin D alone. Further studies by Dawson-Hughes et al. (1997) and Larsen et al. (2004) have also demonstrated a reduction in fracture incidence in older people living in the community. However, this consistency has not been maintained in two recent studies in the UK. A randomized controlled trial of calcium and vitamin D supplementation for fracture prevention in women aged over 70 years, living in the community, was unable to show any beneficial fracture-reduction risk from supplementation (Porthouse et al. 2005). In addition, the large Medical Research Council's RECORD (Randomised Evaluation of Calcium OR vitamin D) trial of calcium and/or vitamin D in the secondary prevention of osteo-porotic fractures has failed to find any benefit from calcium alone, vitamin D alone or combined supplementation when compared with placebo (RECORD Trial Group 2005):

- Randomized controlled trial in 5292 women or men aged over 70 with low-trauma fracture.
- Treated with vitamin D and placebo, calcium and placebo, vitamin D and calcium or double placebo.
- Outcome measures: fractures, morbidity, 25(OH)D, PTH, BMD and falls.
- No reduction in risk of fracture or falls.
- Findings do not support routine supplementation with calcium and vitamin D, either alone or in combination, for the prevention of further fractures in previously mobile elderly people.

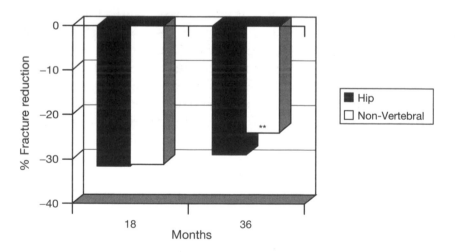

Figure 4.4 Calcium and vitamin D and fracture prevention.

Vitamin D

Vitamin D is essential for skeletal health, maintaining calcium homeostasis via its action at the level of the intestine and bone. Exposure to sunlight and the subsequent cutaneous production of vitamin D_3 is the major source of this vitamin with only about 10% being derived from the diet. Ergocalciferol (vitamin D_2) is the form of vitamin D found in plants and yeast, and cholecalciferol (vitamin D_3) is the form found in oily fish, fish liver oils, margarine and other fat spreads. These dietary forms of vitamin D are fat-soluble substances that are primarily absorbed from the proximal small bowel and transported through the lymphatic system. All sources of vitamin D are biologically inert until they undergo successive hydroxylation in the liver and kidney.

Various groups in the UK are especially vulnerable to vitamin D deficiency; increased skin pigmentation and reduced sunlight exposure (as a result of strict dress codes) expose infants, young children and pregnant women of Asian, African and African–Caribbean origin to the risk of developing vitamin D deficiency. Strict vegans, who eat no meat or oily fish, may also be prone to vitamin D deficiency. From a dietary perspective, individuals with malabsorption syndromes or those who have undergone extensive gastric surgery may be at risk of vitamin D insufficiency. Low bone density may be associated with coeliac disease, particularly in the presence of vitamin D deficiency (Fickling et al. 2001). Two prospective studies have shown that fracture risk is increased in Crohn's disease (Jahnsen et al. 2002), consistent with findings of vitamin D deficiency associated with this condition. Additional individuals who may need vitamin D supplementation include those who are on anticonvulsant therapy, individuals taking rifampicin and those with nephrotic syndrome.

Vitamin D deficiency is common in elderly people (Figure 4.5), particularly those with hip fracture, when more than half of these patients may be vitamin D deficient. Contributory factors are poor nutrition, decreased synthesis of vitamin D_3 and reduced exposure to sunlight. Vitamin D deficiency in elderly people contributes to osteoporosis and fractures through its effects, not only through bone fragility but also by impaired muscle strength, which increases the likelihood of falls in elderly people (Janssen et al. 2002).

A number of preparations of vitamin D and its metabolites are available but there is uncertainty as to the best dose and route of administration. The benefits of supplementing this group of people

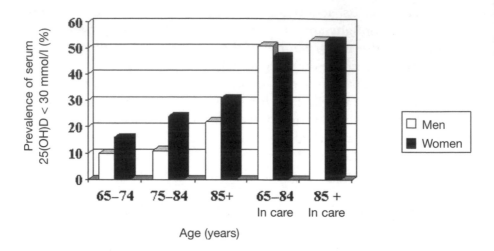

Figure 4.5 Vitamin D status in older people in the UK. 25(OH)D, 25-hydroxyvitamin D. (From Finch et al. 1998.)

with vitamin D alone remain controversial, with clinical studies yielding inconsistent results and little effect on hip fracture reduction. A Finnish study demonstrated that an annual intramuscular injection of 150 000–300 000 IU vitamin D decreased the overall risk of fractures in elderly people by 25% (Heikinheimo et al. 1992). In contrast, a Norwegian study demonstrated no effect of vitamin D 400 IU daily on hip or non-vertebral fractures in 1144 nursing home residents (Meyer et al. 2002). A recent study showed an overall reduction in fractures of 22% with 100 000 IU vitamin D_3 every 4 months in 2037 men and 649 women aged 65–85 years (Trivedi et al. 2003). This result only just achieved statistical significance and the study was inadequately powered to examine the effect of treatment on hip fractures. A British study from 2004 of more than 9000 elderly men and women has shown that an annual intramuscular injection of vitamin D (300 000 IU) was not effective in preventing hip and other non-vertebral fractures (Smith et al. 2004).

Based on the currently available evidence, high levels of dietary calcium are likely to enhance the accrual of bone in prepubertal children and thereby increase peak bone mass; continued on a life-long basis dietary calcium intake will potentially afford some protection against fractures. Calcium and vitamin D supplementation may prevent bone loss and reduce the incidence of hip fractures in frail elderly people and may improve muscle tone, thus reducing the risk of falls.

Dietary alkali

The benefit of a high intake of fruit and vegetables, and hence a high intake of dietary alkali, on skeletal integrity has gained prominence in the literature over a number of years (Barzel 1995). Natural states of acid loading/acidosis have been associated with negative calcium balance and the detrimental effects of acid from the diet on bone mineral have been demonstrated (Arnett 2003). Several population-based studies have shown a beneficial effect of fruit and vegetable/potassium intake on bone mass and bone metabolism in men and women across the age ranges. Further recent support for a positive link between fruit and vegetable intake and bone health can be found in the results of the DASH (Dietary Approaches to Stopping Hypertension) intervention trial (Appel et al. 1997, Lin et al. 2003). The results of DASH 1 showed that an increased intake of fruit and vegetables had a positive effect on calcium economy, with further benefits on the skeleton being demonstrated in the DASH 2 study. Although further research is needed to determine the long-term impact of the DASH diet on bone health and fracture risk, it would appear wise to promote a high intake of fruit and vegetables across all age ranges.

Other nutritional factors

Vitamins A, C, B and K are all potentially important in determining bone health but many of the data on these individual nutrients are sparse, usually observational and based on small studies only. In particular low dietary intake of vitamin K (found in green leafy vegetables, some vegetable oils and fermented foods such as cheese) is associated with low BMD and increased risk of fracture (Booth 2003). Two long-term intervention trials with vitamin K supplementation (Bolton-Smith et al. 2001, Braam et al. 2003) have been completed, both trials suggesting that the combination of vitamin K and vitamin D significantly improves BMD and reduces the rate of bone loss. A number of leading experts have formulated the consensus opinion that a minimal daily intake between 200 and 500 µg/day of vitamin K may be the lower level for optimal bone health (Vermeer et al. 2004). As vitamin K from supplements generally shows a better bioavailability, similar benefits may be achieved by supplements providing an extra dose of 100 mg/day.

Zinc, copper, manganese and boron all have a plausible biochemical basis for influencing bone health but there is only limited information relating to possible independent effects on bone health of these nutrients. Zinc is known to affect infant growth through either indirect mechanisms or direct effects on bone. A positive association has been noted between higher intakes of zinc and bone density in middle-aged premenopausal women. One small trial in healthy postmenopausal women demonstrated a positive effect on spine bone density when zinc was combined with calcium, manganese and copper (Strause et al. 1994).

Studies examining the effects of fluoridation of drinking water on fracture rates have proved inconclusive, although the duration of studies may be too short to demonstrate such an effect (McDonagh et al. 2000). Although studies do not support water fluoridation for the prevention of osteoporosis, nor do they suggest any detrimental effect on the skeleton.

It is suggested that carbonated drinks or beverages containing caffeine are detrimental to bone health, but it is difficult to assess this effect because high caffeine intake is often associated with other risk factors. High caffeine has been associated with decreased BMD in postmenopausal women who have low calcium intakes; however, other studies of peri- and postmenopausal women have found no association between caffeine intake and bone density. Carbonated soft drinks are a popular consumption among the adolescent population, and McGartland and colleagues (2003) demonstrated that high consumption of these drinks in females may impair optimization of peak bone mass.

Phytoestrogens

Phytoestrogens, which are widely distributed within the plant kingdom, are functionally similar to 17β-estradiol. Of particular importance to the human diet are the isoflavones and the lignans, which are found in high concentrations in legumes (soy products) and grains, cereals and linseed, respectively. The growing interest in phytoestrogens is based on epidemiological data, which suggest that populations consuming phytoestrogen-rich diets have a lower incidence of atherosclerotic disease, breast, endometrial and colon cancers, osteoporosis and menopausal symptoms. The incidence of osteoporosis is lower in Asian women than in their western counterparts, and Japanese women have been reported to have a lower incidence of hip fracture than white women. Six studies have assessed the relationship between dietary soy intake and BMD in the Japanese population, with three of these finding a positive correlation (Nagata et al. 2002). Four short-term (6-month) studies on the effects of different isoflavone preparations on BMD in humans have been undertaken (Albertazzi 2002). These have shown a possible beneficial effect on bone density, while taking isoflavones, but any long-term effect is uncertain. Unfortunately there is a marked lack of standardization of these supplements, with preparations varying in their potency and side effects, so it is difficult to ascertain the true benefits of these preparations.

Smoking

Kanis and colleagues (2005) have confirmed that a history of smoking carries a modest but significant risk for future fractures with the effect of smoking being greater than the effect that can be explained by variations in BMD. Current smoking was associated with a significantly increased risk of any kind of fracture in both men and women, with the effect of smoking waning slowly after a person stops smoking. Bone loss is reported to be higher in male smokers than in female smokers, perhaps as a result of men's higher exposure to cigarette smoking.

There are several mechanisms whereby smoking might adversely affect fracture risk. Female smokers have an earlier menopause and increased rates of bone loss after the menopause, suggesting that smoking may enhance oestrogen catabolism. Smokers are also thinner and hence have a lower body mass index; consequently the protective effect of adipose tissue and peripheral oestrogen metabolism is impaired.

Alcohol

Although the influence of modest alcohol intake on the skeleton is uncertain, it potentially affects calcium metabolism and may lead to reduced bone density. Heavy alcohol consumption is associated with a reduction in bone density and increased fracture risk. There is probably a direct effect of ethanol on osteoblasts, but in addition relative malnutrition, lack of exercise and impaired vitamin D metabolism will increase the likelihood of osteoporosis and fractures.

Exercise

Physical activity, particularly weight-bearing exercise, provides the mechanical stimulus or 'loading' important for the maintenance and improvement of bone health, whereas physical inactivity has been implicated in bone loss and its associated health costs (Snow et al. 1996). The impact of exercise is caused by gravitational factors or muscle pull-producing strains within the skeleton, which are perceived by bone cells as osteogenic. Repetitive weight-bearing exercise (e.g. jumping) imposes the necessary strains, strain rates and unusual strain distributions. Skeletal loading also arises from the pull of contracting muscles attached to bone, with muscles having to generate high forces, in order to achieve body movement and lifting. As a result of this, resistance exercise (or weight training) can also have the desired effects (Figure 4.6). Optimal physical activity produces enough strain to maintain or improve bone strength, although the activity needs to be within safe limits; unless it is more than customary it will not produce improvements, e.g. extra walking, at a normal pace, in excess of 10 minutes daily has failed to increase BMD at vulnerable sites for fracture (Martin and Notelovitz 1993).

The starting age of activity is important, with the benefit to bone being doubled if the activity is commenced before or at puberty (Kannus et al. 1995). In adulthood, exercise appears largely to preserve bone rather than add new bone and, in the immediate postmenopausal years, it is unlikely that exercise will balance the effect of oestrogen deficiency. Exercise can improve gait, balance, coordination, proprioception, reaction time and muscle strength in elderly people and subsequently decrease the risk of falls. It can also

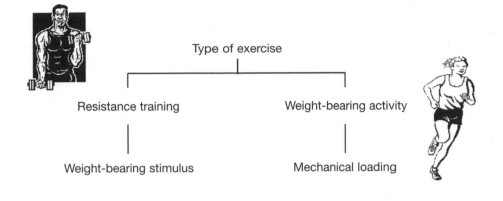

Type of exercise

Resistance training   Weight-bearing activity

Weight-bearing stimulus   Mechanical loading

Figure 4.6 Exercise and prevention of osteoporosis.

lift depression and mood and help with urinary urgency.

The most compelling evidence for a beneficial effect of exercise on BMD is during skeletal growth. However, these effects are difficult to study because of the variability in bone maturation from region to region, with children of a similar chronological age not being at a similar stage of skeletal or sexual maturation. In childhood, moderate exercise appears to increase BMD in both girls and boys (Morris et al. 1997, Bradney et al. 1998). Gymnastics that provides brief and varied skeletal stimulation is effective with evidence that prepubertal gymnasts will have higher BMD than age-matched controls (Bass et al. 1998). Furthermore Kannus and colleagues (1995) have reported bilateral differences in bone mass two to four times higher in tennis players who started training before menarche, compared with those who started 15 years after menarche. Jumping may also be highly effective and one study suggests that in prepubertal children the benefits outlast the intervention (Fuchs et al. 2002). In view of these findings, it is important that young children be encouraged to participate in varied activities throughout their early lives.

The anabolic effect of exercise is less in the adult than in the child, with moderate exercise having little effect in increasing bone mass. Cross-sectional and longitudinal studies with pre- and postmenopausal women have led to inconsistent findings, partly explained by the small sample sizes of published studies, differences in population characteristics, sites and outcomes studied, and differences in experimental designs.

Several meta-analyses of the effects of physical activity have suggested that aerobic exercise and weight training may result in small increases in bone density of about 2%. A meta-analysis in 1997 (Berard et al. 1997), covering 18 randomized and non-randomized studies, confirmed that moderate intensity exercise programmes had a beneficial effect on spinal BMD, in healthy postmenopausal women. Similar results were found by Wolff and colleagues in 1999, demonstrating consistency in the spine and hip in pre- and postmenopausal women. Analysis of results from trials on 699 postmenopausal women demonstrated that women who exercised increased lumbar spine BMD by 1%, compared with controls whose BMD declined by 1% over the same period of time (Kelley et al. 2002). However, a further recent meta-analysis was unable to demonstrate the efficacy of resistance training on increasing or maintaining lumbar spine and femoral neck BMD in premenopausal women (Kelley and Kelley 2004). In older women over the age of 65 years, randomized intervention studies assessing the effects of brisk walking, weight-bearing, and strength and resistance training have suggested that exercise may prevent or slow bone loss by a small amount, particularly in the spine.

It is uncertain how long the benefits of exercise, pursued during young adulthood, will last with advancing years. Studies on those participating in different sports, e.g. tennis and football, have suggested lasting benefits until the late 60s, but it is likely that this benefit will last only if there is continued activity at lower levels for the remainder of life.

Although there has never been a randomized trial showing that exercise reduces fracture risk, this lack of evidence is not necessarily lack of efficacy. Various observational and case–control studies have suggested that those with a lower prevalence of past or current physical activity are at increased risk of hip fracture. Daily standing, climbing stairs and walking are activities deemed to be associated with a lower risk of hip fracture in women. In the Study of Osteoporotic Fracture (SOF), a longitudinal study of more than 9000 women, aged over 65 years, those in the highest quintile of current activity had a 42% lower hip fracture risk than the least active quintile (Gregg et al. 1998). In addition there is independently replicated evidence of an association between physical activity in youth and adulthood and lower risk of hip fracture in men (Kujala et al. 2000).

Exercise during growth results in a high peak BMD and higher muscle strength; continued low level exercise may maintain some of the benefit, but dose–response relationships need to be quantified as do the effects of exercise on bone size, shape, architecture, muscle function and fall frequency. Specific exercise training programmes may be worth considering in the prevention of osteoporosis, but doubts remain about the practicalities of this approach. The beneficial effects probably persist only for the duration of exposure to exercise and the dropout rate from organized exercise programmes is high (Gleeson et al. 1990). Furthermore, the maximum length of programmes reviewed is only 2 years, highlighting the need for studies of a longer duration to evaluate the feasibility and relevance of the use of exercise for bone preservation.

The most common lifestyle interventions that have been examined with respect to the maintenance of skeletal health are the effects of calcium and vitamin D intake, tobacco consumption and exercise. Nutrition is a modifiable factor that is amenable to change and also has important public health implications. It is important that sensible and simple nutritional advice, based on sound scientific evidence, is given throughout life. During childhood and adolescence dietary calcium intake will enhance peak bone mass and, at the other end of the age spectrum, calcium and vitamin D have been shown to be effective strategies for fracture prevention in frail elderly people.

As physical exercise is readily available, relatively cheap and safe, it could represent a cost-effective way of preventing osteoporosis and fractures within the general population. Recommendations for exercise can be made and are generally positive; however, most are opinion and not evidence based. In addition, to achieve maximum benefits on the skeleton demands lifelong adherence and acceptability, which in turn will be determined by the individual's inclination.

References

Albertazzi P (2002) Soy in the prevention of bone loss. Osteopor Rev 10: 1–5.
Appel LJ, Moore TJ, Obarzanek E et al. (1997) A clinical trial of the effects of dietary patterns on blood pressure. N Engl J Med 336: 1117–24.

Arnett T (2003) Regulation of bone cell function by acid-base balance. Proc Nutr Soc 62: 511–20.

Barzel US (1995) The skeleton as an ion exchange system: Implications for the role of acid–base balance in the genesis of osteoporosis. J Bone Miner Res 10: 1431–6.

Bass S, Saxon L, Daly R (1998) Heterogeneity in the osteotrophic response to physical loading during different stages of puberty. J Bone Miner Res 15(suppl 1): 558.

Berard A, Bravo G, Gauthier P (1997) Meta analysis of the effectiveness of physical activity for the prevention of bone loss in postmenopausal women. Osteopor Int 7: 331–7.

Bolton-Smith C, Mole PA, McMurdo MET et al. (2001) Two year intervention study with phylloquinone (vitamin K), vitamin D and calcium: Effect on bone mineral content. Ann Nutr Metab 45(suppl 1): 246.

Bonjour JP, Chevalley T, Ammann P, Slosman D, Rizzoli R (2001) Gain in bone mineral mass in prepubertal girls 3.5 years after discontinuation of calcium supplementation: A follow-up study. Lancet 358: 1208–12.

Booth S (2003) Dietary vitamin K and skeletal health. In: New SA, Bonjour JP (eds), Nutritional Aspects of Bone Health. Cambridge: Royal Society of Chemistry, pp. 323–38.

Braam LA, Knapen MH, Geusens P et al. (2003) Vitamin K supplementation retards bone loss in postmenopausal women between 50 and 60 years of age. Calcif Tissue Int 73: 21–6.

Bradney M, Pearce G, Naughton G et al. (1998) Moderate exercise during growth in prepubertal boys: Changes in bone mass, size, volumetric density and bone strength: A controlled prospective study. J Bone Miner Res 13: 1814–21.

Chapuy MC, Arlot ME, Duboeuf F et al. (1992) Vitamin D and calcium to prevent hip fractures in elderly women. N Engl J Med 327: 1637–42.

Chapuy MC, Arlott ME, Delmas PD, Meunier PJ (1994) Effect of calcium and cholecalciferol treatment for 3 years on hip fracture in elderly women. BMJ 308: 1081–2.

Cummings SR, Nevitt M, Browner W et al. (1995) Risk factors for hip fracture in white women. N Engl J Med 332: 767–73.

Dawson-Hughes B, Harris SS, Krall EA, Dallal GE (1997) Effect of calcium and vitamin D supplementation in men and women 65 years of age or older. N Engl J Med 337: 670–6.

Fickling WE, MacFarlane XA, Bhalla AK, Robertson DA (2001) The clinical impact of metabolic bone disease in coeliac disease. Am J Gastroenterol 96: 112–19.

Finch S, Doyle W, Lowe C et al. (1998) National Diet and Nutrition Survey. London: The Stationery Office.

Francis RM (1996) Prevention and treatment of osteoporosis: Calcium and vitamin D. In: Compston JE (ed.), Osteoporosis. New perspectives on causes, prevention and treatment. London: Royal College of Physicians of London, pp. 123–34.

Francis RM, New SA (2003) Book review: Understanding, preventing and overcoming osteoporosis by Plant J & Tidey G. Osteopor Rev 11(4): 11.

Fuchs RK, Snow CM, Marcus R (2002) Gains in hip bone mass from high impact training are maintained: A randomised controlled trial in children. J Pediatr 141: 357–62.

Gillespie WJ, Avenell A, Henry DA, O'Connell DL, Robertson J (2004) Vitamin D and vitamin D analogues for preventing fractures associated with involutional and post-menopausal osteoporosis (Cochrane Review). In: The Cochrane Library, Issue 1. Chichester: John Wiley & Sons Ltd.

Gleeson PB, Protas E, LeBlanc A, Schneider VS, Evans HJ (1990) Effects of weight lifting on bone mineral density in pre menopausal women. J Bone Miner Res 5: 153–8.

Gregg EW, Cauley JA, Seeley DG et al. (1998) Physical activity and osteoporotic fracture risk in older women. Study of Osteoporotic Fractures Research Group. Ann Intern Med 129: 81–8.

Heaney RP (2000) Calcium, dairy products and osteoporosis. J Am Coll Nutr 19(2 suppl): 83S–99S.

Heaney RP (2002) The importance of calcium intake for lifelong skeletal health. Calcif Tissue Int 70(2): 70–3.

Heikinheimo RJ, Inkovaara JA, Harju EJ et al. (1992) Annual injection of vitamin D and fractures of aged bones. Calcif Tissue Int 51: 105–10.

Iuliano-Burns S, Saxon L, Naughton G, Gibbons K, Bass SL (2003) Regional specificity of exercise and calcium during skeletal growth in girls: A randomised trial. J Bone Miner Res 18: 156–62.

Jahnsen J, Falch JA, Mowinckel P, Aadland E (2002) Vitamin D status, parathyroid hormone and bone mineral density in patients with inflammatory bowel disease. A population based cohort study. Ann Intern Med 133: 795–9.

Janssen HC, Samson MM, Verhaar HJ (2002) Vitamin D deficiency, muscle function and falls in elderly people. Am J Clin Nutr 75: 611–15.

Johnell O, Gullberg B, Kanis JA et al. (1995) Risk factors for hip fracture in European women: The MEDOS study. J Bone Miner Res 10: 1802–15.

Kanis JA, Johnell O, Oden A et al. (2005) Smoking and fracture risk: A meta-analysis. Osteopor Int 16: 155–62.

Kannus P, Haapasalo H, Sakelo M et al. (1995) Effect of starting age of physical activity on bone mass in the dominant arm of tennis and squash players. Ann Intern Med 123: 27–31.

Kelley GA, Kelley KS (2004) Efficacy of resistance exercise on lumbar spine and femoral neck bone density in premenopausal women: A meta analysis of individual patient data. J Women's Health 13: 293–300.

Kelley GA, Kelley KS, Tran ZV (2002) Exercise and lumbar spine bone mineral density in post menopausal women: A meta analysis of individual patient data. J Gerontol Biol Sci Med Sci 57: 599–604.

Kujala UM, Kaprio J, Kannus P et al. (2000) Physical activity and osteoporotic hip fracture risk in men. Arch Intern Med 160: 705–8.

Larsen ER, Mosekilde L, Foldspang A (2004) Vitamin D and calcium supplementation prevents osteoporotic fractures in elderly community dwelling residents: A pragmatic population based three year intervention study. J Bone Miner Res 19: 370–8.

Lin PH, Ginty F, Appel L et al. (2003) The DASH diet and sodium reduction improve markers of bone turnover and calcium metabolism in adults. J Nutr 133: 3130–6.

McDonagh MS, Whiting PF, Wilson PM, Sutton AJ, Chestnutt I, Cooper J (2000) Systematic review of water fluoridation. BMJ 321: 844–5.

McGartland C, Robson PJ, Murray L et al. (2003) Carbonated soft drink consumption and bone mineral density in adolescence: The Northern Ireland Young Hearts Project. J Bone Miner Res 18: 1563–9.

Martin D, Notelovitz M (1993) Effects of aerobic training on bone mineral density of post menopausal women. J Bone Miner Res 8: 931–6.

Matkovic V, Crnevic-Orlic Z, Landoll J (2003) Role of calcium in maximising peak bone mass development. In: New SA, Bonjour JP (eds), Nutritional Aspects of Bone Health. Cambridge: Royal Society of Chemistry, pp. 129–44.

Meyer HE, Smedshaug GB, Kvaavik E, Falch JA, Tverdal A, Pedersen JI (2002) Can vitamin D supplementation reduce the risk of fracture in the elderly? A randomized controlled trial. J Bone Miner Res 17: 709–15.

Morris FL, Naughton GA, Gibbs JL et al. (1997) Prospective ten month exercise intervention in premenarcheal girls: Positive effects on bone and lean mass. J Bone Miner Res 12: 1453–62.

Nagata C, Shimizu H, Takami R et al. (2002) Soy product intake and serum isoflavones and oestradiol concentration in relation to bone mineral density in postmenopausal women. Osteopor Int 13: 200–4.

Plant J, Tidey G (2003) Understanding, Preventing and Overcoming Osteoporosis. London: Virgin Books Ltd.

Porthouse J, Cockayne S, King C et al. (2005) Randomised controlled trial of calcium and supplementation with cholecalciferol (vitamin D_3) for prevention of fractures in primary care. BMJ 330: 1003–6.

RECORD Trial Group (2005) Oral vitamin D_3 and calcium for secondary prevention of low trauma fractures in elderly people (Randomised Evaluation of Calcium Or vitamin D, RECORD): A randomized placebo controlled trial. Lancet (online): DOI:1016/S0140–6736(05)63013–9.

Smith H, Andeson F, Raphael H et al. (2004) Effect of annual intramuscular vitamin D supplementation on fracture risk. Osteopor Int 15(suppl 1): S8.

Snow CM, Shaw JM, Matkin CC (1996) Physical activity and risk for osteoporosis. In: Marcus R, Feldman D, Kelsey J (eds), Osteoporosis. San Diego, CA: Academic Press, pp. 511–28.

Specker BL (2000) Should there be a dietary guideline for calcium intake? No. J Am Coll Nutr 71: 661–4.

Strause L, Saltman P, Smith KT, Bracker M, Andon MB (1994) Spinal bone loss in postmenopausal women supplemented with calcium and trace minerals. J Nutr 124: 1060–4.

Trivedi DP, Doll R, Khaw KT (2003) Effect of four monthly oral vitamin D3 (chole-calciferol) supplementation on fractures and mortality in men and women living in the community: Randomised double blind controlled trial. BMJ 326: 469–72.

Vermeer C, Shearer MJ, Zitterman A et al. (2004) Beyond deficiency: Potential benefits of increased intakes of vitamin K for bone and vascular health. Eur J Nutr 43: 325–35.

Wolff I, Van Croonenborg JJ, Kemper HCG et al. (1999) The effect of exercise training programs on bone mass: A meta analysis of published controlled trials in pre and post menopausal women. Osteopor Int 9: 1–12.

CHAPTER 5

Diagnosis of osteoporosis

- Bone mineral density (BMD) measurements by dual energy X-ray absorptiometry (DXA) at the spine and hip are the current 'gold standard' for the diagnosis of osteoporosis and intervention with treatment
- Bone mineral density measured by DXA is strongly related to fracture risk
- If DXA is not available, measurements at peripheral sites, combined with risk factor assessment, may be useful in predicting fracture risk
- Bone markers may indicate progressive bone loss and, in addition to DXA, may strengthen the indication for treatment and also monitor response to therapy
- Risk assessment with or without BMD will help to predict absolute fracture risk

This chapter describes the current techniques that are available for measuring bone density, their mode of operation, the nature of their results and their ability to predict fracture risk. It also explores the value and clinical utility of clinical risk assessment.

Bone densitometry is a generic term denoting the non-invasive measurement of bone microarchitecture to predict its strength. A variety of modalities are in current use, including dual energy X-ray absorptiometry (DXA) and peripheral X-ray absorptiometry (PIXI), and the use of electromagnetic radiation in quantitative computed tomography (QCT). High-frequency sound waves are used in ultrasound measurements of bone and over the last decade research into the role of magnetic resonance (MR) has shown that it has potential as a useful method for evaluating bone microstructural information as well as bone density.

In clinical practice, DXA is currently the most widely used and it is generally accepted that it is the 'gold standard' for the measurement of bone mineral density (BMD). It has advantages of good precision, short scan times and stable calibration in clinical use. It allows scanning of the spine and hip, usually regarded as the most important measurement sites because they are common types of osteoporotic fractures resulting in morbidity and mortality (Figure 5.1).

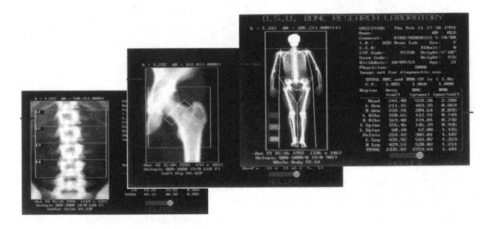

Figure 5.1 Dual energy X-ray absorptiometry (DXA): reporting.

Dual energy X-ray absorptiometry integrates the measurement of all the bone structures in the path of a scanning beam including cortical and trabecular bone into one value (Figure 5.2). Beams of radiation at two energy levels generated from an X-ray source are scanned across the bone in a two-dimensional fashion. The detector measures the attenuation of the two beams and, by integrating the relative attenuation of the low- and high-energy beams, it is able to define the bone area and subtract attenuation caused by soft tissue from the bone image. By dividing the bone mineral content (BMC) by the bone area, a third measurement, the BMD, is derived and is expressed in grams per square centimetre. Different DXA machines have been calibrated against standards that differ in size and composition so those comparisons of machine values in grams per square centimetre are not valid. To overcome these problems, bone density values are commonly expressed in standard deviation units with reference to either the

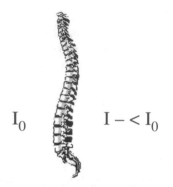 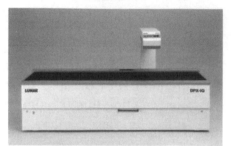

$$I_0 \qquad I - < I_0$$

Measures narrow beam of X-rays
transmitted through bone

Figure 5.2 Dual energy X-ray absorptiometry (DXA): mode of action.

age-matched range (Z score) or the young normal range consisting of individuals at peak bone mass (T score). These methods of expressing the bone density value are valid because bone density values at a particular age have a normal distribution.

The lower the bone density T or Z scores the higher the risk of fracture. In age-related and postmenopausal osteoporosis the relative risk of fracture rises by about twice for each standard deviation below normal, irrespective of age and gender. For the purpose of clinical decision-making, a World Health Organization (WHO) study group recommended a definition of osteoporosis based on BMD measurements of the spine, hip or forearm expressed as T scores (WHO 1994). This definition was originally developed for white women and suggested that a woman with a T score below −2.5 at the spine, hip or forearm had osteoporosis; the term 'osteopenia' was used if the T score was between −2.5 and −1. This level was chosen because it defined the lower limit of normal in relation to the young healthy skeleton and also because it selected individuals at high risk of fracture. This definition cannot automatically be applied to other BMD measurement sites or to other technologies such as QCT or quantitative ultrasonography (QUS). Further studies of the applicability of the WHO criteria to men are required, although studies show a similar relationship between BMD and fracture risk in both sexes, suggesting that they may also be applicable to men. The use of T scores in young adolescents and children is inappropriate but work is ongoing in the UK to establish good quality reference data for specific use within the field of paediatric DXA (Crabtree et al. 2004).

Although DXA is currently the best available clinical method for the prediction of bone fragility, it does have some limitations. It reflects BMC but is unable to measure bone structure and volumetric bone mineral distribution, which are also fundamental determinants of bone strength and fracture risk. There are also inherent inaccuracies in DXA that arise from technical constraints and, before any scan is reported, it requires careful scrutiny.

Whether scanning patients to identify those with low bone mass or monitoring response to treatment, it is important that bone density measurements are performed at sites that respond quickly to changes in skeletal status and where the benefits of therapy can be measured after a reasonably short time. For many applications, the lumbar spine has proved the ideal site because of the metabolically active trabecular bone in the vertebral bodies. The spine is routinely scanned in the posteroanterior position but more modern DXA systems are able to perform lateral spine measurements. The advantage of this technique is that the vertebral body can be isolated and evaluated without the influence of osteophytes that will distort the image. With the advent of higher-resolution DXA systems, visual assessment of fractures is also possible from DXA-based lateral spine images. Compared with a conventional spine radiograph, DXA may provide clearer visualization of fractures, can also measure vertebral heights and involves much less radiation. This technique does not, however, identify other potential problems that would be apparent on a plain spine radiograph; it requires more elaborate positioning of the patient, more specialized skills from the operator and currently would not be a surrogate for a spine radiograph. A careful scrutiny of the scan image is important in the interpretation of DXA studies to ensure that anatomical and other artefacts do not affect the findings, e.g. degenerative disease and vertebral fractures will spuriously elevate the results, noticeably at individual vertebral levels. In elderly individuals in particular the spine scan may be of little value if there is marked degenerative disease.

When the hip is scanned, measurements are given for the femoral neck, greater trochanter, Ward's triangle and total hip. Geometric measurements of the hip have been developed and incorporated into the DXA scanning software; importantly the hip axis length has been identified as an independent indicator of hip fracture risk and this is obtainable from a standard DXA scan. The hip can also show a range of anatomical variants that may impede accurate measurement, including Paget's disease of the hip, marked osteoarthritis and incorrect rotation or abduction of the leg. For patients who have had hip replacement surgery, most DXA machines have special software available to measure the bone density around the metal implant. In this way, bone loss around the implant can be detected and it is hoped that this might provide an early indicator of implant failure.

It is also possible to perform DXA measurements of the forearm, although this is not usually offered as part of a routine scan. Scanning covers the distal half of the forearm from the midradius to the wrist, with measurements recorded for the radius and ulna either separately or combined. This site may be useful for monitoring rates of change in cortical bone.

The clinical indications for performing BMD measurements have been summarized by the Royal College of Physicians' guidelines (1999). In addition a DXA scan should be performed only if it is going to influence a decision on treatment.

Follow-up DXA scans may be offered depending on resources. These are performed to monitor response to treatment and it is believed that they may enhance patient compliance with long-term therapy. The appropriate interval between serial BMD scans is determined from the concept of the 'least significant change' in BMD. For any changes in BMD to be true, the measured change must exceed 2.8 times the precision error. Patel et al. (2000) have reported long-term precision errors of 1.6% for the spine and total hip BMD, thereby producing a figure of 4.5% for the least significant change. As it is unlikely that such a significant change in BMD will be detectable in less than 2 years, BMD scans are normally not repeated more frequently than every 2 years. Ideally repeat scans should be performed on the same machine using the same scan mode. A visual comparison should be made with previous scans and the patient's weight needs to be checked because major weight change can affect the scan result because of changes in body fat.

Indications for DXA

Early menopause
Amenorrhoea
Male hypogonadism
Oral steroid therapy
Other secondary causes
Osteopenia on radiograph
Previous fragility fracture
Maternal history of hip fracture
Low body mass index (BMI 19 kg/m^2)
Loss of height, kyphosis
Vertebral deformities on radiograph

Peripheral DXA

Peripheral devices that use DXA technology (Figure 5.3) are available for scanning the forearm and calcaneus. These devices are cheaper and smaller, and therefore require less room and are potentially portable. They are relatively simple to operate but, as they still deliver

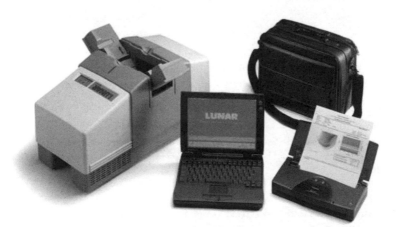

Figure 5.3 Peripheral dual energy X-ray absorptiometry.

low doses of radiation, compliance with appropriate radiation regula-
tions is still essential. Results are reported in terms of BMC, BMD, and
T and Z scores. A major disadvantage of this technique is the varied reference data provided by the different manufacturers of these systems.
There are variations in the size, sex, age distribution and racial mix of
the population on which the normal reference range is based. There
is a paucity of appropriate reference data for children and racial
groups other than white people, and only limited data for men and
premenopausal women. In view of these failings, peripheral devices
are not totally reliable in diagnosing osteoporosis.

Various studies have, however, shown that peripheral devices may
predict future fracture risk (Marshall et al. 1996, Miller et al. 2002).
Used in conjunction with a clinical risk assessment, results from
peripheral devices may be useful as part of a triage approach to the
management of osteoporosis. It has been suggested that, once upper
and lower thresholds have been established for individual systems, it
would be possible tentatively to diagnose osteoporosis in those with a
low T score, whereas those above the higher threshold would be
unlikely to have osteoporosis (Table 5.1). Those between the lower
and upper thresholds would require a central DXA measurement to
confirm the absence or presence of osteoporosis. A recent study has
confirmed the theoretical expectation that implementation of this
algorithm would require around 40% of women to be referred for central DXA measurements (Blake et al. 2004).

Table 5.1 Peripheral bone measurements

For	Against
Rapid and clear imaging	Not site specific
Predicts fracture risk	Cannot monitor response
Easy to use	
Cheap at £20 000	
→ Portable	
Low PIXI → ? BMD	
Low PIXI + Strong risk factors → ? Treat	

BMD, bone mineral density; PIXI, peripheral X-ray absorptiometry.

Ultrasonography

Measurement of bone by QUS has been available for many years; although it has been widely researched, its use in clinical practice remains restricted. QUS is measured by assessing the passages of sound waves through or along bone to measure several parameters. There are three basic types of QUS scanner: two methods measure mainly trabecular bone using a transmission method, whereas the third uses a reflective method and measures cortical bone. The transmission method uses either a water- or dry-based contact system and is restricted to measurements at the calcaneus. The reflective method is used largely at the phalanges, radius and tibia, all sites of cortical bone. Although QUS cannot be used to diagnose osteoporosis, its use has been shown to be predictive of fractures, particularly in elderly people, and for hip fractures. The EPIDOS study, a large prospective trial of the risk of hip and other fractures in France, demonstrated that QUS was able to predict hip fracture risk in elderly women as well as DXA (Hans et al. 1996).

Studies investigating the use of QUS in a clinical setting show that there is probably a strong case for using QUS as another risk factor alongside existing clinical risk factors. QUS may therefore be useful in an area where access to DXA is limited or as part of a triage system. Although there are some data showing the predictive capacity of QUS parameters for fracture in men, there is little evidence to support its use in adolescents or young children. The combination of limited precision and the slow rate of change of bone mass at appendicular sites means that it is difficult to use QUS to monitor response to treatment and this approach is not recommended.

Quantitative computed tomography

Quantitative computed tomography is the only truly three-dimensional bone mass measurement technique available. It has the unique ability to differentiate cortical and trabecular bone, and may be used clinically to measure the bone density of the spine. At the hip there is currently no standard QCT protocol for assessing BMD, but several researchers have explored the application of QCT to model the complex geometry of the proximal femur. At present the use of QCT is limited in the clinical setting as CT scanners are more expensive than DXA scanners, the precision of the BMD measurements is poorer and the radiation dose to the patient is much higher.

Magnetic resonance

Magnetic resonance is a complex technique based on the use of high magnetic fields, transmission of radiofrequency (RF) waves and the detection of RF waves from the region being scanned. With respect to assessing bone microarchitecture, two approaches have been developed: indirect assessment of trabecular structure from studies of the MR relaxation times of the adjacent bone marrow (MR relaxometry) and direct assessment of trabecular structure by high-resolution imaging of trabecular bone (MRI).

At the current level of knowledge MR relaxometry is an exciting research tool for investigating the role of microstructural deterioration in osteoporosis and the effects of therapy in modifying this risk. Its role in clinical practice is, however, unproven, primarily as a result of the limited data demonstrating its utility in the prediction of fracture risk. The ability of MRI to provide structural information on trabecular bone is a powerful research tool for understanding the interrelationship of bone density, microstructure and fracture risk. Studies examining this technique in clinical practice are still preliminary, but in the future MR may play a routine clinical role and refine the selection of patients for more aggressive therapy to prevent fracture.

Bone markers

The level of bone mass can be assessed with adequate precision by measuring BMD using DXA; however, this measurement does not capture all risk fractures for fracture. Bone fragility also depends on the morphology, the architecture and the remodelling of bone as well as on the quality (properties) of the bone matrix, which can be readily assessed. Evidence accumulated over the last few years has suggested that bone strength may be reflected independently of BMD level, by measuring bone turnover using specific serum and urinary markers of bone formation and resorption. Bone turnover markers have also been suggested as useful in monitoring the efficacy of treatment with antiresorptive (hormone replacement therapy, bisphosphonates, calcitonin) and anabolic agents (parathyroid hormone).

Bone remodelling is the result of two opposing activities: the production of new bone matrix by osteoblasts and the destruction of old bone by osteoclasts. These rates of production and destruction can be evaluated either by measuring predominantly osteoblastic or osteclastic enzyme activities or by assaying bone matrix components released into the bloodstream and excreted in the urine. Although these have been separated into markers of formation and resorption, in osteoporosis where both events are coupled any marker will reflect the overall rate of bone turnover. At present, in serum, the most sensitive markers for bone formation are serum osteocalcin, bone alkaline phosphatase and procollagen type N-terminal propetide (PINP). For the evaluation of bone resorption, immunological assays of pyridinium cross-links of collagen have become the best option. Immunological assays are now available for deoxypyridinoline (DPD) in urine and for C-terminal and N-terminal type collagen peptides (CTX and NTX) in serum or urine (Table 5.2).

Table 5.2 Biochemical markers

Formation	Resorption
Measured in serum	*Measured in serum and urine*
Osteocalcin (OC)	C-terminal (S-CTX) cross-linking telopeptide of type I collagen (serum)
Bone alkaline phosphatase (ALP)	Deoxypyridinoline (DPD)
Procollagen type I C+N propeptide (PICP + PINP)	N-terminal (U-NTX) + C-terminal (U-CTX) cross-linking telopeptide of type I collagen (urine)

Bone markers and fracture risk prediction

Previous work by Garnero and colleagues (1996) suggested that one of the important applications of bone turnover markers in osteoporosis was to predict fracture risk in postmenopausal women. These findings were then confirmed by other prospective studies that consistently reported that bone resorption assessed by urinary or serum CTX or urinary free deoxypyridinoline above the premenopausal range is associated with about a twofold higher risk of hip, vertebral and non-hip and non-vertebral fractures over follow-up periods ranging from 1.8 years to 5 years (Garnero 2000). More recently it has been shown that increased levels of urinary osteocalcin also predicted the risk of clinical vertebral fractures in a large prospective study of elderly women (Gerdhem et al. 2004). The identification of prospective fracture patients is one of the key goals in osteoporosis; this may be aided by the use of bone markers in addition to BMD measurements and other risk factors. The combinations of bone markers with other diagnostic tests, including BMD, should be validated in further prospective studies of postmenopausal women and operational thresholds should be developed and adapted to treatment strategies. The value of bone turnover markers for the prediction of fracture risk in other populations, such as men, also needs to be explored in large and long-term studies.

Bone markers and treatment monitoring

Monitoring the efficacy of treatment of osteoporosis is a challenge. The goal of treatment is to reduce the occurrence of fragility fractures, but a low incidence of fractures and the absence of events during the initial years of therapy do not necessarily imply that the treatment is effective. Although BMD may be used for monitoring response to treatment, the response is slow and it usually takes at least 2 years for BMD to exceed the least significant change. DXA does not allow the identification of all responders within the first year of therapy. Bone markers indicate early treatment effects on bone metabolism. A decrease in bone resorption markers is rapid after starting treatment, with maximum suppression of bone resorption markers of about 50% occurring within 3 months of starting antiresorptive treatment. The effect on bone formation markers is seen at 6 months and after this time bone turnover is stabilized at a lower level. It is presumed that the early identification of a response to treatment may aid patient compliance; should no response be found this raises the question of patient adherence and also the problem of genuine failure to respond to therapy.

The principal disadvantages to using bone turnover markers to monitor therapy are their variability, the inconvenience of sample collection and their cost. Blood samples can be taken any time but urine specimens should be collected at the same time on each occasion.

There are strong indications that biochemical markers may add an independent, predictive value to the assessment of bone loss and fracture risk. There are also potential advantages for monitoring the effects of treatment, particularly to identify non-responders or non-compliance by individuals. Currently they are used widely as research tools or clinically in specialist centres but their transition into everyday clinical practice may be fast approaching.

Risk assessment

Although BMD measurements have previously been used to ascertain the need for treatment there is growing recognition that these alone will not predict absolute risk of fracture. There are a large number of risk factors that are consistently associated with fracture risk.

Because osteoporosis is basically asymptomatic, we need to identify those patients who may be osteoporotic *before* a fracture occurs.

Risk assessment

Early menopause
Low trauma fracture
Oral steroids
Other causes of secondary osteoporosis
Low BMI
Smoking
Family history of hip fracture

Apart from age, sex and geographical location, risk factors include prior fractures, use of glucocorticoids, low BMI and certain diseases associated with osteoporosis. Other putative risk factors such as family history of fracture and smoking require wider validation. The importance of these risk factors differs: some act independently, others dependently and yet others are partially dependent. There are several considerations in the selection of risk factors for use in fracture prediction because different risk factors have different relevance at different ages, e.g. an early menopause is a significant risk factor for any osteoporotic fracture in perimenopausal women, but is of uncertain significance for fracture in elderly women. Conversely, a family history of hip fracture appears to be a risk factor in elderly women, but is not a consistent risk factor at menopause. Different risk factors may also have different relevance for varied fracture sites, e.g. high BMI and smoking are risk factors for ankle fractures but these factors do not contribute significantly to the risk of forearm fractures at the same age. It is thus evident that risk factor assessment needs to consider age and distribution of fracture types, along with other variously weighted risk factors. The clinical risk factors used for fracture prediction should be selected with care and validated in multiple populations. They should be adjusted for age and type of fracture, be readily assessable by all health-care professionals, contribute to a risk that may be modified by therapeutic manipulation and be intuitive to medical care.

The Swedish Council on Technology Assessment in Health Care (SBU 2003) has performed the most extensive and systematic review of osteoporosis and has graded the evidence concerning various risk factors. This work, which has drawn on 14 databases from around the

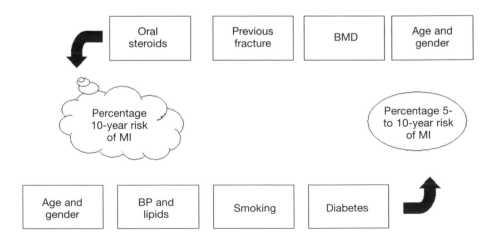

Figure 5.4 Fracture risk assessment. MI, myocardial infarction; BP, bisphosphonate.

world, is still ongoing. In the future it is envisaged that there will be an algorithm for risk assessment leading to absolute probability of fracture and subsequent need for intervention. This has been likened to the management of cardiovascular disease when there is simultaneous consideration of smoking, blood pressure, diabetes and serum cholesterol, which permits the identification of patients at high risk (Figure 5.4). Once this algorithm has been developed it is anticipated that it will help to target the correct individuals at highest absolute risk of fracture.

Current clinical evaluations of osteoporosis and the assessment of bone fragility rely largely on DXA and, particularly, on its primary outcome BMD measured at the spine or hip. Of the variety of central and peripheral methods, central DXA is still considered to be the clinical standard for the diagnosis of osteoporosis and related research. It is, however, clear that the use of DXA does not capture all risk factors for fracture with bone fragility, depending also on bone morphology, architecture, rate of remodelling and quality of bone matrix. The use of bone markers is increasingly valid in these areas and in the future the ideal measurement of skeletal integrity may include both the use of DXA and markers in the clinical arena. In addition, it is clear that an understanding of clinical risk factors along with knowledge of bone density is necessary to achieve a prediction of future fracture probability.

References

Blake GM, Chinn D, Steel S, Patel R, Panayioyou E, Fordham J (2004) The revised NOS position statement on peripheral x ray absorptiometry: A listing of device specific thresholds for the clinical interpretation of PDXA examinations. Osteopor Int 15(suppl 2): S15.

Crabtree NJ, Oldroyd B, Truscott JG et al. (2004) UK paediatric DXA reference data (GE Lunar Prodigy): Effects of ethnicity, gender and pubertal status. Osteopor Int 15(suppl 2): 10.

Garnero PP (2000) Markers of bone turnover for the prediction of fracture risk. Osteopor Int 11(suppl 6): S55–65.

Garnero P, Hausherr E, Chapuy MC et al. (1996) Markers of bone resorption predict hip fracture risk in elderly women: The EPIDOS Prospective Study. J Bone Miner Res 11: 1531–8.

Gerdhem P, Ivaska KK, Alatalo SL et al. (2004) Biochemical markers of bone metabolism and prediction of fracture in elderly women. J Bone Miner Res 19: 386–93.

Hans D, Dargent-Molina P, Schott AM et al. (1996) Ultrasonographic heel measurements to predict hip fracture in elderly women: The EPIDOS prospective
study. Lancet 348: 511–14.

Marshall D, Johnell O, Wedel H (1996) Meta analysis of how well measures of
bone density predict occurrence of osteoporotic fractures. BMJ 312: 1254–9.

Miller PD, Siris ES, Barrett-Connor E et al. (2002) Prediction of fracture risk in
postmenopausal white women with peripheral bone densitometry: Evidence
from the National Osteoporosis Risk Assessment. J Bone Miner Res 17:
2222–30.

Patel R, Blake GM, Rymer J, Fogelman I (2000) Long term precision of DXA scanning assessed over seven years in forty postmenopausal women. Osteopor Int
11: 68–75.

Royal College of Physicians (1999) Osteoporosis: Clinical guidelines for prevention and treatment. London: RCP.

Swedish Council on Technology Assessment (SBU) (2003) Osteoporosis:
Prevention, diagnosis, treatment. Report No. 165, vols 1 and 2. Stockholm:
SBU.

World Health Organization (1994) Assessment of Facture Risk and Its Application
to Screening for Postmenopausal Osteoporosis. Technical Report Series 843.
Geneva: WHO.

CHAPTER 6

Treatment of osteoporosis

- There is an expanding range of treatment options available for preventing bone loss and fractures
- The National Institute for Health and Clinical Excellence (NICE) has recently published guidance on the use of bisphosphonates, raloxifene and teriparatide in the secondary prevention of osteoporotic fractures
- Long-term adherence to therapy remains inconsistent

There are now a number of effective treatments for osteoporosis that increase bone density and reduce the incidence of fractures. These drugs can be broadly divided into antiresorptive and anabolic agents. The former inhibit osteoclast activity, decrease bone resorption and, because of the transient uncoupling of bone turnover, result in a modest increase in bone mineral density (BMD) of between 5 and 10%, predominantly in the first year of treatment. In contrast anabolic agents work by increasing bone formation and can lead to greater increases in BMD by up to 50%. Strontium ranelate is the first in a new class of drugs – dual acting bone agents (DABAs) – that increases bone formation and reduces bone resorption. Antiresorptive treatments commonly used include bisphosphonates, raloxifene, calcitonin and hormone replacement therapy (HRT). In the clinical setting teriparatide is the one drug that has an anabolic effect.

In considering the choice of treatment in the individual patient a number of factors are important, including the underlying pathogenesis of bone loss, evidence of efficacy in any particular situation, the cost of treatment, tolerability and patient preference. Past guidance on treatment was issued by the Royal College of Physicians in 1999 and subsequently updated in 2000 (RCP 1999, 2000). Using an evidence-based approach the treatment recommendations in Table 6.1 were

Table 6.1 Treatment of osteoporosis

Treatment	Vertebral fracture	Hip fracture
Hormone replacement therapy	A	B
Raloxifene	A	N/D
Etidronate	A	B
Alendronate	A	A
Risedronate	A	A
Teriparatide	A	N/D
Calcium/Vitamin D	N/D	A

Evidence from A: randomized controlled trials, B: other controlled trials and epidemiological studies. N/D, trials not done. Adapted from RCP and BTSGB Guidelines (2000).

Table 6.2 NICE Technology Appraisal Guidance 87: secondary prevention of fragility fractures

Bisphosphonates	Raloxifene	Teriparatide
Recommended in:	Second-line treatment option for women in whom:	In women aged > 65 years, who have had an inadequate clinical response or intolerance to BPs and are at quadrupled risk of further fracture:
Women aged > 75 years, without DXA	Bisphosphonates are contraindicated	T score < –4.0 on DXA
Women aged 65–75 years, with T score < –2.5, confirmed by DXA	Unable to comply with instructions	Two or more recent fractures and a very low BMD (T score < –3.2) and another risk factor
Women < 65 years if they are at doubled risk for another fracture: T score < –3.0 on DXA T score < –2.5 and low BMI (< 19 kg/m²), current smoker, maternal hip fracture, systemic steroids or condition affecting bone	Inadequate clinical response	
	Intolerance of bisphosphonates	

BMD, bone mineral density; BMI, body mass index; BPs, bisphosphonates; DXA, dual energy X-ray absorptiometry. T score is the bone density value commonly expressed in standard deviation units with reference to the young normal range consisting of individuals at peak bone mass.

made. The National Institute for Health and Clinical Excellence (NICE) has recently completed a Health Technology Appraisal on bisphosphonates, raloxifene and teriparatide. Guidance on their use in the secondary prevention of fragility fractures in postmenopausal women who have already sustained a clinically apparent osteoporotic fracture is now available (Table 6.2). Further recommendations will be made on the use of these drugs with respect to primary prevention and strontium ranelate will also be subject to a technology appraisal by 2006.

Bisphosphonates

Bisphosphonates are the most commonly used antiresorptive agents in the treatment of osteoporosis. Cyclical etidronate (Didronel PMO) was the first bisphosphonate to be licensed in the UK and, although still available, its use has now been largely superseded by alendronate (Fosamax) and risedronate (Actonel). Most studies of alendronate and risedronate have been performed in postmenopausal women but Gonnelli and colleagues (2003) also demonstrated favourable long-term effects of alendronate in men with overall effects on BMD similar to those seen in women. Bisphosphonates are also the most effective agents for managing glucocorticoid-induced osteoporosis (Amin et al. 2002).

Both alendronate and risedronate can be taken on a once-daily basis but in an attempt to improve patient convenience and long-term adherence to treatment, and to reduce potential gastrointestinal complications that may be associated with daily use, once-weekly regimens have also been developed. These regimens provide the sum of seven daily doses of alendronate (70 mg weekly) and risedronate (35 mg weekly) and are pharmacologically equivalent to the daily doses.

Bisphosphonates concentrate exclusively in the skeleton by suppressing osteoclast-mediated bone resorption at the surface of bone. After exerting their action, they become embedded in bone where they remain, biologically inert, for a long period of time. With the resumption of bone resorption in these areas, bisphosphonates will be released from bone and excreted in the urine, but their metabolic fate locally is unknown. In all clinical studies reported so far there have been no safety concerns with their use for up to 10 years. However, because of their long residence time in bone and their ability to suppress bone resorption, their long-term safety with respect to bone tissue has been queried. Reassuringly recent dog studies have demonstrated that very high doses of bisphosphonates given for a long time to a non-osteoporotic animal model do not compromise bone strength (Burr et al. 2003).

Administration of alendronate and risedronate decreases the rate of bone turnover, increases BMD at relevant skeletal sites, and significantly reduces the risk of vertebral and non-vertebral fracture. Spine bone density in women with osteoporosis is increased by 5–8% over 2–3 years, with an approximate 60% reduction in the incidence of further vertebral fractures (Harris et al. 1999, Black et al. 2000) (Figure 6.1). Risedronate and alendronate also increase hip bone density by 4.1–5.9% in 3 years and effectively reduce the incidence of other non-vertebral fractures (Harris et al. 1999, Black et al. 2000) (Figure 6.2). Systematic reviews with meta-analyses have shown that the anti-fracture efficacy of these two bisphosphonates is consistent among trials and populations.

As bisphosphonates are poorly absorbed, the timing and mode of administration is critical: etidronate must be taken at least 2 hours before or after food, whereas alendronate and risedronate should ideally be taken at least 30 min before the first food of the day. Bisphosphonates may cause mild gastrointestinal disturbance; to avoid this the medication needs to be taken with a large glass of water and recumbency avoided after administration. Severe oesophagitis occurs rarely, usually if the patient is non-compliant with the recommended instructions or has a past history of upper gastrointestinal disease. Other noted side effects may be joint pains and occasional skin reactions. The complex instructions for the administration of bisphosphonates may limit adherence with treatment, particularly in unsupervised patients with cognitive impairment. Although the introduction of weekly preparations of alendronate and risedronate improves the convenience of bisphosphonate treatment for many patients, some find it easier to remember to take them on a daily basis.

Intermittent intravenous administration of bisphosphonates may help to solve the problems of long-term adherence and gastrointestinal intolerance experienced with the oral bisphosphonates. In clinical trials zolendronate, given at intervals of up to 1 year, has produced

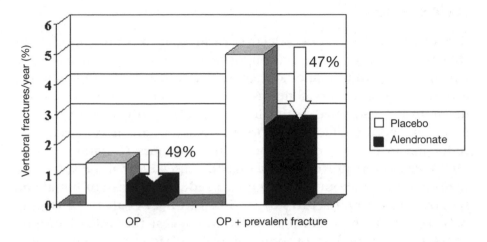

Figure 6.1 Effect of alendronate on vertebral fractures. OP, osteoporosis. (From Black et al. 2000.)

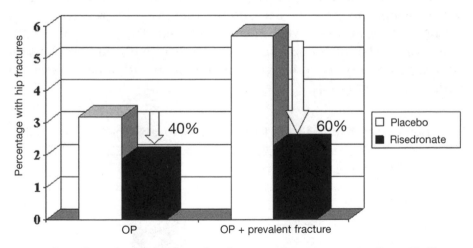

Figure 6.2 Effect of risedronate on hip fractures. OP, osteoporosis. (From McClung et al. 2001.)

comparable effects on bone density and fracture incidence as oral dosing (Reid 2002). Ibandronate is another new preparation undergoing clinical trials; it may be given orally every month or intravenously every 2–3 months and appears to produce beneficial effects on BMD and fracture incidence (Wasnich Adami and Viapiana 2003).

Raloxifene

Raloxifene (Evista) is a selective oestrogen receptor modulator (SERM). This type of drug has opposite activities in specific tissues as a result of the conformational changes that it makes on binding to the estradiol receptor. Raloxifene has agonist actions on the skeleton, acting as an antiresorptive agent without exhibiting any bone toxicity. Its major antagonist effect is on breast tissue, where it can lead to a reduction in oestrogen-receptor-positive tumours (Cummings et al. 1999). Raloxifene prevents bone loss, increases BMD at the spine and femoral neck by about 2–3%, and also reduces the risk of initial and recurrent vertebral fractures by 30–50% (Ettinger et al. 1999) (Figure 6.3). However, there is no evidence to suggest that raloxifene prevents the risk of hip or other peripheral fractures. Taken as a once-daily preparation, raloxifene is generally well tolerated with mild side effects including leg cramps and swelling of the hands and feet. Given to the early postmenopausal woman it can cause vasomotor symptoms and its use should therefore be reserved for a woman who is at least 1 year postmenopausal. There is also a slightly increased risk of venous thromboembolism with this preparation so it is potentially contraindicated in a woman with a past history of deep vein thrombosis.

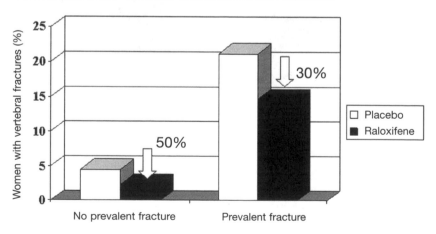

Figure 6.3 Raloxifene and vertebral fractures. (From Ettinger et al. 1999.)

Calcitonin

Calcitonin is a potent antiresorptive agent with a rapid but short-lived effect on osteoclast function. Calcitonin is a naturally occurring polypeptide hormone, usually secreted by the parafollicular cells of the thyroid; the source of pharmacological calcitonin is salmon or human. It can be given either subcutaneously or intranasally with various dosing regimens and frequency of administration. Early studies of parenteral calcitonin in postmenopausal women with osteoporosis showed small increases in BMD and a reduction in vertebral fractures (Rico et al. 1992). The PROOF (Prevention of Occurrence of Osteoporotic Fractures) study investigated the effects of 5 years' intranasal calcitonin (Miacalcic) in 1255 women with osteoporosis (Chesnut et al. 2000). Treatment with calcitonin resulted in a modest increase in BMD; although the 200 IU dose significantly reduced the risk of new vertebral fractures by 33%, the decrease in fractures with 100 and 400 IU was not statistically significant. There are no serious side effects with calcitonin use, but they may include flushing, vomiting, diarrhoea and local irritation when injected, or nasal crusting or secretion when taken intranasally. In view of the relatively poor data on anti-fracture efficacy, calcitonin should probably be used only in patients who are unable to tolerate other treatments.

Calcitonin may, however, be very useful in the acute management of vertebral fractures where it appears to confer analgesic properties. The exact mechanism of pain control is not known, but it has been hypothesized that calcitonin stimulates endorphin release. Given both nasally and subcutaneously it leads to a reduction in pain within 2 weeks and subsequent improvement in mobility. These beneficial effects appear to persist for at least 4 months without any marked side effects (Maksymowych 1998).

Hormone replacement therapy

Hormone replacement therapy (HRT) comprises treatment with oestrogen, with the addition of cyclical or continuously administered progestogen, in women who have not been hysterectomized. Both prospective cohort studies and large randomized clinical trials have demonstrated its efficacy in terms of prevention of postmenopausal bone loss. It has been found that low doses of oestrogens are effective and that the route of administration does not influence this effect. Past small studies of HRT demonstrated its effectiveness in reducing the incidence of vertebral and non-vertebral fractures (Lufkin et al. 1992, Komulainen et al. 1998). A more recent meta-analysis has suggested a 33% reduction in vertebral fracture and a 27% decrease in non-vertebral fracture incidence (Torgerson and Bell-Syer 2001). Findings from the USA, from the Women's Health Initiative (WHI – a series of large clinical trials), have confirmed the beneficial effects of continuous combined oestrogen and progestogen on fracture outcomes (Rossouw et al. 2002) (Figure 6.4). However, this arm of the WHI study was curtailed after 5 years as a result of the excess number of breast cancer cases; in addition, those using HRT were also shown to have a higher incidence of coronary events, strokes and pulmonary emboli. On the basis of these findings, continuous combined HRT is no longer recommended as a long-term therapy for the prevention of bone loss or treatment of established disease in older women. The WHI oestrogen-only trial was continued until February 2004 and again demonstrated a beneficial effect of oestrogen on the skeleton. This preparation did not affect coronary heart disease rates but did increase the risk of stroke.

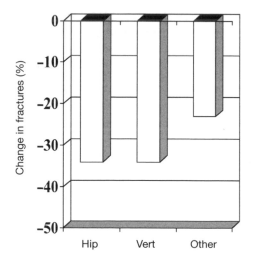

Figure 6.4 Women's Health Initiative HRT study. (From Rossouw et al. 2002.)

Unexpectedly, women taking oestrogen alone appeared to have a lower risk of developing breast cancer compared with those women taking a placebo, although the estimated 7 fewer cases per 10 000 person-years did not reach statistical significance (WHI Steering Committee 2004). Women taking oestrogen only can be reassured that there is no excess risk of heart disease or breast cancer for at least 6 years of use, but they need to be counselled about the increased stroke risk. HRT remains effective in preventing fracture in the younger postmenopausal woman (Randell et al. 2002), and should climacteric symptoms also be present it may be worth considering this form of treatment for a relatively short period of time at the smallest effective dose.

Teriparatide

Teriparatide (Forsteo) is recombinant human parathyroid hormone 1–34 and is the first licensed anabolic treatment for osteoporosis. Parathyroid hormone (PTH) is secreted from the four parathyroid glands and regulates calcium and phosphate metabolism in the bones and kidneys. Chronic elevation of PTH results in a greater degree of bone resorption and thus depletion of calcium, leading to osteoporosis. In contrast, intermittent pharmacological administration of PTH has the seemingly paradoxical effect of increasing bone mass, so reducing programmed cell death (apoptosis) of osteoblasts and osteoclasts, and thus prolonging their survival. It also exerts a number of other effects on bone cells, accounting for its anabolic activity although, for most of these effects, the mechanism of action at the level of molecular physiology remains largely unknown. Currently, teriparatide is given daily as a subcutaneous injection over a period of 18 months and then discontinued; the effects of a longer-term course of treatment on bone mass and fracture risk remain uncertain. The first randomized, placebo-controlled clinical trial to establish vertebral and non-vertebral fracture efficacy studied the effects of teriparatide in 1637 postmenopausal women with osteoporosis (mean age 69 years). This study showed that 21 months' treatment with daily subcutaneous injections increased BMD by 9–13% more in the lumbar spine and 3–6% more in the femoral neck when compared with placebo (Neer et al. 2001) (Figure 6.5).

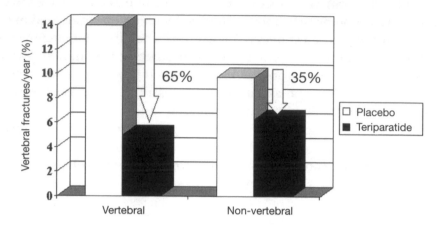

Figure 6.5 Effect of teriparatide on fractures. (From Neer et al. 2001.)

There was also a 65% reduction in new vertebral fractures and a 53% reduction in non-vertebral fractures. It has been hypothesized that the administration of teriparatide simultaneously with bisphosphonates could enhance the effect on bone mass. However, studies by Finkelstein et al. (2003) and Black et al. (2003) have concluded that there is no reason to combine alendronate and teriparatide, and that the addition of alendronate may actually impair the anabolic activity of PTH on trabecular bone tissue. It also remains to be established whether teriparatide remains effective in patients previously treated with bisphosphonates.

The most common adverse effects associated with teriparatide treatment include nausea, headache and leg cramps; as it is administered by injection it also requires reasonable levels of manual dexterity. Teriparatide is much more expensive than other treatment options and, at present in the UK, on a cost-effective basis alone its use has been limited to those who have failed to respond to other treatments and have an exceedingly low BMD.

Strontium ranelate

Strontium ranelate (Protelos) is the first of a new class of treatments for osteoporosis, a dual action bone agent that reduces bone resorption and increases bone formation. Strontium was investigated for the management of osteoporosis in the 1950s but it was then abandoned because its use was associated with mineralization defects. The poor absorption of strontium chloride taken orally has been overcome by combining the element with ranelate. Although the precise mechanism of strontium ranelate is unknown, it is taken up by calcified tissues, mostly at the surfaces of the bone matrix without affecting mineral structure. At the cellular level it appears to activate the calcium-sensing receptor, consequently inducing osteoblast differentiation. A randomized controlled trial of strontium ranelate (2 g/day) in 1649 postmenopausal women with osteoporosis and at least one vertebral fracture showed increases in BMD of 12.7% in the lumbar spine and 8.6% in the hip after 3 years' treatment, with a 41% reduction in the incidence of new vertebral fracture (Meunier et al. 2004) (Figure 6.6).

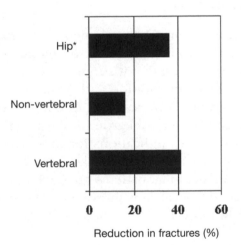

Reduction in fractures (%)

Figure 6.6 Effect of strontium ranelate on fracture reduction. (From Meunier et al. 2004.)

It must be noted, however, that about 50% of this apparent increase is spurious, caused by the skeletal incorporation of strontium, which has a higher atomic number than calcium. There is also evidence suggesting that strontium may reduce the incidence of non-vertebral fractures. In a study of 5901 women with osteoporosis a 16% reduction in the incidence of non-vertebral fractures overall was noted, but in a subgroup analysis in 1977 women aged over 74 years with low BMD (T score < −3.0), the hip fracture risk was reduced by 36% (Rizzoli et al. 2004). Strontium ranelate is available in powder form in sachets, the contents of which are dissolved in water. It should preferably be taken at bedtime, at least 2 hours after eating, to ensure optimal absorption from the bowel. Strontium has been well tolerated in clinical trials, with no evidence of an increase in upper gastrointestinal side effects; diarrhoea has been reported in a small number of patients but this appears to be short-lived (Meunier et al. 2004). Strontium is now available in the UK and is likely to be useful in the management of older women with osteoporosis, particularly those unable to tolerate bisphosphonates.

Calcium and vitamin D

The role of calcium and vitamin D supplementation, particularly in frail elderly people, has already been covered in Chapter 4. In addition there is some evidence to suggest that it should be co-prescribed with bisphosphonates, raloxifene, teriparatide and strontium. These drugs are all effective in preventing bone loss but in clinical trials this has been demonstrated only against a background of calcium and vitamin D repletion, and the UK licence indications for these therapies stipulate that adequate calcium and vitamin D intake should be maintained. Unless the clinician is confident that patients are calcium and vitamin D replete, it is recommended that calcium and vitamin D supplementation should be considered in those patients where there is a possibility of insufficiency.

Adherence to treatment

Lack of adherence to long-term treatments for chronic conditions is an important issue. Among other factors patient adherence is governed by beliefs about the severity of the patient's illness and relevant treatment. Illness-related factors include severity of symptoms, level of disability and rate of progression. Treatment-related factors include complexity and duration of treatment regimen, immediacy of beneficial effects, and perceived or actual side effects. Despite studies showing that osteoporosis treatments are generally well tolerated and associated with significant efficacy benefits, adherence to therapies is generally poor. Of patients taking a once-daily bisphosphonate, 77% stop treatment within a year with almost two-thirds of patients taking a once-weekly preparation also failing to adhere to treatment (DIN-LINK 2004). This, in part, may be a result of the fact that treatments need to be taken long term and are not associated with any short-term symptomatic benefits.

In addition the dosing regimen of some preparations is slightly complex and all treatments may give rise to side effects. Adherence rates to osteoporosis treatment will also be influenced by other concomitant medications – a particular problem with advancing age when over 50% of people aged over 70 take three or more prescribed medicines. Non-adherence to osteoporosis treatments has significant repercussions for a patient's prognosis, with evidence showing greater fracture reduction in those who adhere to therapy compared with those who do not (Caro et al. 2004). In attempting to compare adherence rates to daily or weekly dosing with bisphosphonates, it has been suggested that adherence to weekly preparations is better but still needs substantial improvement (Cramer et al. 2004, Recker et al. 2004). On initiation of therapy, it is important that patients be advised on mode of administration and side effects. Most treatments for osteoporosis will need to be taken long term and some patients may require reviews to check their adherence to therapy.

Several new drug targets for osteoporosis have recently been identified and it is anticipated that they will provide the basis for new therapies in the future. These largely represent novel molecular mechanisms involved in regulating osteoblast function and generation. Other studies have also suggested that it may be possible to develop further drugs that enhance osteoblast survival by inhibiting apoptosis (Tobias and Hickey 2004).

At present there is the option of treating patients with several drugs that demonstrate good fracture reduction levels. These include bisphosphonates, raloxifene, HRT, PTH and strontium. Indications for pharmaceutical intervention are mainly based on BMD measurements, with reference for treatment determined by WHO criteria. Prior fracture history and additional risk factors and glucocorticoid use have also been included in various guidelines and appraisals. Pertinent strategies are, however, still required to identify all those who require therapy. In addition, the unresolved problem surrounding long-term adherence for some patients still requires attention.

References

Amin S, Lavalley MP, Simms RW, Felson DT (2002) The comparative efficacy of drug therapies used for the management of corticosteroid induced osteoporosis: A meta regression. J Bone Miner Res 17: 1512–26.

Black DM, Thompson DE, Bauer DC et al. (2000) Fracture risk reduction with alendronate in women with osteoporosis: The Fracture Intervention Trial. FIT Research Group. J Clin Endocrinol Metab 85: 4118–24.

Black DM, Greenspan SL, Ensrud KE et al. (2003) The effects of parathyroid hormone and alendronate alone or in combination in post menopausal osteoporosis. N Engl J Med 349: 1207–15.

Burr DB, Miller L, Grynpas M et al. (2003) Tissue mineralisation is increased following 1 year treatment with high doses of bisphosphonates in dogs. Bone 33: 960–9.

Caro J, Ishak KJ, Huybrechts KF, Raggio G, Maujocks C (2004) The impact of compliance with osteoporosis therapy on fracture rates in actual practice. Osteopor Int 15: 1003–8.

Chesnut CH, Silverman S, Andriano K et al. (2000) A randomised trial of nasal spray salmon calcitonin in postmenopausal women with established osteoporosis: The prevent recurrence of osteoporotic fractures study. Am J Med 109: 267–76.

Cramer JA, Amonkar MM, Hebborn A, Suppapanya N (2004) Does dosing regimen impact persistence with bisphosphonate therapy among postmenopausal women? J Bone Miner Res 19(suppl 1): S448.

Cummings SR, Eckert S, Krueger KA et al. (1999) The effect of raloxifene on risk of breast cancer in postmenopausal women: Results from the MORE randomised trial. Multiple Outcomes of Raloxifene Evaluation. JAMA 281: 2189–97.

DIN-LINK (2004) Osteoporosis Report 4, All diagnoses. CompuFile Ltd.

Ettinger B, Black DM, Mitlak BH et al. (1999) Reduction of vertebral fracture risk in postmenopausal women with osteoporosis treated with Raloxifene. Results from a 3 year randomised clinical trial. JAMA 282: 637–45.

Finkelstein JLS, Hayes A, Hunzelman JL, Wyland JJ, Lee H, Neer RM (2003) The effects of parathyroid hormone, alendronate, or both in men with osteoporosis. N Engl J Med 349: 1216–26.

Gonnelli S, Cepollaro C, Montagnani A et al. (2003) Alendronate treatment in men with primary osteoporosis: A three year longitudinal study. Calcif Tissue Int 73: 133–9.

Harris ST, Watts NB, Genant HK et al. (1999) Effects of risedronate treatment on vertebral and non vertebral fractures in women with postmenopausal osteoporosis: A randomised controlled trial. Vertebral Efficacy with Risedronate Therapy (VERT) Study Group. JAMA 282: 1344–52.

Komulainen MH, Kroger H, Tuppurainen MT et al. (1998) HRT and Vit D in prevention of non-vertebral fractures in postmenopausal women: A 5 year randomized trial. Maturitas 31: 45–54.

Lufkin EG, Wahner HW, O'Fallon WM et al. (1992) Treatment of post-menopausal osteoporosis with transdermal oestrogen. Ann Intern Med 117: 1–9.

McClung MR, Geusens P, Miller PD et al. (2001) Effect of risedronate on the risk of hip fractures in elderly women. Hip Intervention Study Group. N Engl J Med 344: 333–40.

Maksymowych WP (1998) Managing acute osteoporotic vertebral fractures with calcitonin. Can Fam Physician 44: 2160–6.

Meunier PJ, Roux C, Seeman E et al. (2004) The effects of strontium ranelate on the risk of vertebral fracture in women with postmenopausal osteoporosis. N Engl J Med 350: 459–68.

Neer RM, Arnaud CD, Zanchetta JR et al. (2001) Effect of parathyroid hormone (1–34) on fractures and bone mineral density in postmenopausal women with osteoporosis. N Engl J Med 344: 1434–41.

Randell KM, Honkanen RJ, Kroger H, Saarikoski S (2002) Does hormone replacement therapy prevent fractures in early postmenopausal women? J Bone Miner Res 17:528–33.

Recker RR et al. (2004) Medication persistence is better with weekly bisphosphonates but it remains suboptimal. J Bone Miner Res 19 (suppl 1): 5172.

Rico H, Henandez ER, Revilla M, Gomez-Castresana F (1992) Salmon calcitonin reduces vertebral fracture rate in post menopausal crush fracture syndrome. Bone Miner 16: 131–8.

Rizzoli R, Reginster JY, Diaz-Curiel M et al. (2004) Patients at high risk of hip fracture benefit from treatment with strontium ranelate. Osteopor Int 15(suppl 1): S18.

Rossouw JE, Anderson GL, Prentice RL et al. (2002) Writing Group for the Women's Health Initiative Investigators. Risks and benefits of oestrogen plus progestin in healthy postmenopausal women: Principal results from the Women's Health Initiative randomized controlled trial. JAMA 288: 321–33.

Royal College of Physicians (1999) Osteoporosis: Clinical guidelines for prevention and treatment. London: RCP.

Royal College of Physicians of London and Bone and Tooth Society of Great Britain (2000) Clinical Guidelines for Prevention and Treatment. London: Royal College of Physicians.

Tobias J, Hickey S (2004) Emerging therapies for osteoporosis. In: Woolf A, Akesson K, Adami S (eds), The Year in Osteoporosis, Vol. 1. Oxford: Clinical Publishing, pp. 297–318.

Torgerson DJ, Bell-Syer SE (2001) Hormone replacement therapy and prevention of vertebral fractures: A meta-analysis of randomised trials. BMC Musculoskel Dis 2: 7.

Wasnich Adami S, Viapiana O (2003) Ibandronate: New options in the treatment of osteoporosis. Drugs Today 39: 877–86.

Women's Health Initiative Steering Committee (2004) Effects of conjugated equine estrogen in postmenopausal women with hysterectomy. The Women's Health Initiative Randomised Controlled Trial. JAMA 291: 1701–10.

CHAPTER 7

Service provision

- Examples of good practice exist in the UK but provision is haphazard
- Fracture liaison services are central to secondary prevention within secondary care
- Standard 6 of the National Service Framework for Older People suggests that falls and osteoporosis services should be fully integrated
- As a major national health charity, the National Osteoporosis Society offers a large range of services to its members and health-care professionals

Low trauma fractures occurring in older people constitute a major clinical and financial burden to the NHS. In 2002–2003 in the UK there were 78 554 admissions to hospitals for cases of fractured neck of femur. Alongside the hip fractures, there will be significant numbers of patients with other types of fragility fractures. McClellan et al. (2003) have suggested that, for every patient admitted with a hip fracture, there will be three patients treated for a low trauma fracture of the wrist, shoulder, ankle, hand or foot, in addition to uncertain numbers sustaining both symptomatic and silent crush fractures of the spine. Although a number of pharmacological interventions have been shown to prevent further fractures, osteoporosis remains under-diagnosed and many patients do not receive appropriate assessment and management. Studies from the USA in 2003 (e.g. Andrade et al. 2003, Simonelli et al. 2003) demonstrated that osteoporosis was considered as a diagnosis in only 26% of cases and within a year of fracture only a quarter of women had received any treatment for osteoporosis. Within the UK an audit in Sussex in 2003 (Canagon et al. 2003) found that, despite a high profile of osteoporosis in the area, only 6% of patients with a low trauma fracture received a dual energy X-ray absorptiometry (DXA) scan before or after fracture. Only 19% were taking the minimum of the audit standard of vitamin D and/or calcium, and only 3.8% were on antiresorptive agents. A retrospective audit performed in Manchester in 2002 (Charalambous et al. 2002) showed that only 22% of patients aged over 50 admitted to hospital with low trauma fracture and 0% of patients seen in the fracture clinic with distal radius fractures were managed according to osteoporosis guidelines. After the introduction of a protocol for managing osteoporosis in the orthopaedic department, appropriate management rose to 76% in patients with hip fractures and 81% for those with distal radius fractures (Charalambous et al. 2002).

The concept of targeting treatment at those patients most likely to benefit is a central component of osteoporosis management. Patients who have already experienced a fracture are at highest risk of sustaining a further fracture and therefore any intervention that identifies and treats these individuals should be given high priority. The British Orthopaedic Association (BOA) published *The Care of Fragility Fracture Patients* in 2003 (Marsh et al. 2003) and noted the importance of a team approach to secondary prevention of fracture through a dedicated liaison service within a secondary care setting. The aim of this type of service is to optimize selective case finding of patients who have already experienced a fragility fracture, offer them appropriate information on osteoporosis and its management, and provide advice to each patient's GP on suitable pharmacological interventions. This type of service may also provide access to DXA measurements and referral to physiotherapy or falls services when appropriate, and facilitate further investigations if necessary. To identify all patients with fractures, this service would ideally need to liaise among secondary care bone metabolism services, orthopaedic units including fracture clinics and trauma wards, and accident and emergency departments. Developing models of this approach in the UK have found that a dedicated fracture liaison nurse specialist has been pivotal to the success of this service. Experience in the Glasgow Fracture Liaison Service in its first 18 months showed that almost all patients, aged over 50 years, presenting with fragility fracture were identified and assessed (McClellan et al. 2003). Once diagnosed, the continuation of therapy is critical and several studies have shown that those who are seen by a dedicated nurse have a relatively high level of adherence with therapy for up to 3 years after their original consultation (Barton et al. 2003). Although results from these services are encouraging they are not necessarily representative throughout the UK, e.g. data published from Portsmouth showed that only 7% of patients attending fracture clinic were investigated for osteoporosis, with only 18% being prescribed any medication (Shenton et al. 2004). Varied results are also seen with respect to inpatient hip fractures, with Gallagher and colleagues (2004) demonstrating both high levels of prescribing while an inpatient and high levels of adherence after discharge. O'Neill and colleagues (2004), however, reported low levels of ongoing therapy in hip fracture patients once discharged from hospital. These diverse results suggest that there is no room for complacency and that service delivery needs to be continuously developed and refined.

Orthogeriatric provision

The National Service Framework (NSF) for Older People states that 'at least one general ward in an acute hospital should be developed as a centre of excellence for orthogeriatric practice'. It does not, however, recommend a particular type of orthogeriatric collaboration although it advocates that this should be agreed at local level with consideration given to the needs of the service and resources available. There are some data to support the use of orthogeriatric units, in terms of improving likelihood of returning to original place of residence (Cameron et al. 2001). An ideal model should aim to offer continuous combined orthogeriatric care, at both the acute and the rehabilitation phases. Central to the concept of this model is the multidisciplinary team, comprising medical and nursing staff, dietitians, physiotherapists and occupational therapists with well-defined links between primary and secondary care. As many older people who sustain a fracture have associated co-morbidity and diminished physiological reserves, they demand complex medical management on a daily basis.

Early intervention for medical complications is likely to prevent acute deterioration leading to surgical delays or death in the peri- and postoperative period. The period of rehabilitation after surgery depends on the individuals; however, most patients would potentially benefit from some time in a specialist rehabilitation unit. Specialized units have been shown to improve outcomes in stroke but more studies are required to assess the effectiveness of multidisciplinary inpatient rehabilitation for elderly patients with fractures.

Integrated falls and osteoporosis services

The year 2001 saw the publication of the NSF for Older People. Standard 6 set out a standard of care for older people at high risk of falling and recognized that the detection, assessment and care of people with, or at high risk of, osteoporosis was integral to this standard. A key feature of the NSF was the recommendation that integrated services for falls and osteoporosis should be developed and be in place in all local health-care and social care systems by April 2005. It is in the best interests of patients and cost-effectiveness for falls and osteoporosis services to be closely coordinated (Figure 7.1). This is recognized in all the guidelines and applies both to basic risk detection at population level and to the specialized services. Although some of the need can and should be met from better cooperation between existing services, it remains apparent that service delivery has not been maximized on a universal basis.

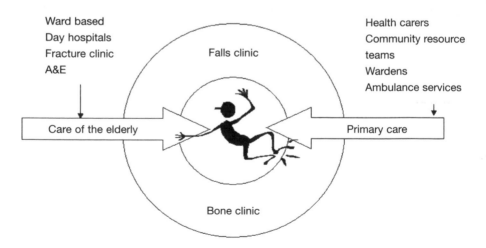

Figure 7.1 Integrating osteoporosis management with falls prevention.

It is doubtful that the interim (2004) target has been universally accomplished and there is concern that full implementation will not take place by April 2005. By 2004 all local delivery plans (LDPs) should have included the development of an integrated falls and osteoporosis service (Figure 7.1). The All Party Parliamentary Osteoporosis Group (APPOG – National Osteoporosis Society or NOS 2004) audited 266 plans and found that 16% of primary care trusts (PCTs) did not contain a reference to either osteoporosis or falls, with 76% of PCTs making no reference to osteoporosis and 17% of PCTs making no reference to falls. Better progress had been made with planning the fall component, but there appeared to be a lack of understanding about the role of osteoporosis in developing an integrated falls service. The findings from the PCTs were also confirmed in the delivery plans of the Strategic Health Authorities (SHAs) with only a third of their plans including an appropriate reference to integrated falls and osteoporosis services. The APPOG has asked a sample of PCTs whether they were likely to meet the April 2005 target, to which 43% have recorded a positive response. Information gathered from the SHAs has suggested that 32% were likely to meet the April 2005 milestone. There are several reasons why service providers have failed to meet the interim target and may fail to reach the 2005 milestone. Information provided by the APPOG's survey suggests that a number of PCTs feel that the government has not prioritized falls and osteoporosis services, this lack of priority being undermined by the exclusion of osteoporosis from the General Medical Service (GMS) contract. In addition, over half of the PCTs believed that a lack of funding, particularly for prescribing and DXA scans, was the main block to implementation. Other identified reasons included the problems associated with multi-agency working when falls and osteoporosis services need to span primary, secondary, social and community care, and issues surrounding staff recruitment.

Despite devolution of the National Health Service (NHS), the APPOG remains convinced that the government has a major role to play in the development of integrated falls and osteoporosis services. Key recommendations include urging the government to incorporate osteoporosis in the GMS contract and to provide leadership and assistance to local health and Social Services to share best practice and interpret national policy at local levels. In turn it is anticipated that this will increase awareness and understanding about the delivery of a fully integrated falls and osteoporosis service.

Nurse-run osteoporosis clinics

The past decade has seen an increase in the number of nurse-run clinics operating in both primary and secondary care. Various catalysts, including response to service development, the extension of the nurse's role and the drive towards collaborative working across traditional boundaries, have prompted their inception. Current social and demographic trends are likely to continue into the foreseeable future, with ageing of the population and the rise in chronic diseases leading to greater demand for health care in both hospitals and the community. At the same time the developments of new technologies will require more practitioners, including nurses, who are able to pioneer new ways of working. In *Making a Difference* (Department of Health 1999), 10 areas of practice were identified that could be undertaken by nurses, provided that they had the appropriate knowledge and training. Key areas relevant to the management of osteoporosis would include the ability of nurses to:

- run their own clinics
- receive referrals from GPs and other clinicians
- make appropriate referrals, e.g. to physiotherapists or pain clinics
- admit and discharge patients within agreed protocols
- request and interpret diagnostic measurements and biochemical profiles investigations, e.g. bone density
- recommend appropriate treatment.

Over the past decade nurse-run osteoporosis clinics have become an integral part of the Metabolic Bone Unit at Freeman Hospital, Newcastle upon Tyne. Historically, patient consultation in the unit was medically dominated, but in response to increasing and changing demands on the service nurse-run clinics were introduced. Referrals to this service are made by the GP or hospital clinician, and they are triaged by the specialist nurse with the patient allocated to either the general metabolic bone clinic or the nurse-run clinic. In general, the patient with a complex medical history or evidence of vertebral fracture is seen in the metabolic bone clinic, whereas the patient with major risk factors for osteoporosis or radiological suspicion of the condition is seen in the nurse-run clinic. Before the clinic visit each patient has bone mineral density (BMD) measurements performed at the spine and hip. With the use of a specifically designed pro forma, information is collected during the consultation. It is envisaged that this approach will be assimilated into a care pathway in the future, collected electronically and stored on a database.

Reasons for referral and brief medical history are recorded. In both sexes, consideration is given to fracture history, presence of back pain, kyphosis and height loss. Attention is focused on current or past steroid use, anticonvulsant use and history of thyroid disease, gastric surgery/disease and frequency of falls. A note is made of a family history of osteoporosis and hip fracture and any other relevant family history. The patient's current medication and known drug allergies are also recorded. A simple analysis is made of the patient's dietary calcium intake, tobacco and alcohol consumption, and levels of exercise. Women are also questioned on current and past menstrual history, age at menopause, use of any hormone replacement therapy (HRT), and history of benign and malignant breast disease, deep vein thrombosis and pulmonary embolus (both personal and familial).

After this assessment the patient is given an explanation of the DXA results which are reported on the pro forma for the attention of the referring clinician. Should the results demonstrate osteoporosis further investigations are performed to identify possible secondary causes, including biochemical profile, thyroid function tests, full blood count, erythrocyte sedimentation rate (ESR), C-reactive protein (CRP) and urinary markers of bone turnover. In addition parathyroid hormone (PTH) and vitamin D estimations are performed in elderly people, with testosterone, sex hormone-binding globulin (SHBG), gonadotrophins and prostate-specific antigen (PSA) being requested in male patients. Should osteoporosis be diagnosed, relevant treatment options are discussed with the patient. Discussion largely focuses on the side effects and mode of administration of bisphosphonates, raloxifene, calcium and vitamin D, strontium and occasionally HRT, calcitonin or teriparatide. The length and complexity of this discussion will depend on the patient's existing knowledge of therapeutic options, preconceptions of osteoporosis and acceptance of the diagnosis. Some patients demonstrate high levels of understanding and are keen to commence treatment immediately, whereas others are uncertain and require more time to consider appropriate options. During the consultation lifestyle issues may be addressed, e.g. dietary calcium intake,

ideal activity levels and falls prevention strategies. All patients are provided with literature on osteoporosis and its treatment, a variety of
leaflets from the National Osteoporosis Society (NOS) and the pharmaceutical industry being used. The concluding section of the pro
forma details a plan of action and makes recommendations for treatment if necessary and appropriate referral to other agencies, e.g.
physiotherapy. Arrangements are made for further review of the
patient, usually after 6 months, to check for adherence to therapy and
for repeat bone density measurements in 2 years' time, where necessary.

Within this nurse-run clinic, the specialist nurse has a high degree
of autonomy but this was achieved only after extensive training in the
management of osteoporosis. The clinic is also part of a consultant-led
metabolic bone service that uses established protocols, evidence-
based guidelines, multidisciplinary working, and formal and informal
pathways of communication. Ideally, the management of osteoporosis
requires a collaborative approach between all health-care professionals in both primary and secondary care. The development of nurse-run
clinics should be considered as one aspect of this approach, but
emphasis must be placed on the structured development of clinics and
rigorous training and education of the nurses involved.

Management of osteoporosis in primary care

There is limited literature showing the likely effect of osteoporosis
on the provision of services at the primary care level. In addition the
absence of standards relating to falls and fractures within the quality
outcomes framework in the contract for GPs tends to negate osteoporosis as a high priority. One example of osteoporosis management
ideally suited to the primary care setting is the use of selective case
finding to identify those at high risk, but this requires refined com-
puter systems, and commitment, enthusiasm and training of primary
care staff. Work completed within the Central Manchester Primary
Care Trust in 2004 (Edlington and O'Brien 2004) highlighted the
variability and quality of data collected between practices, with the
most recent data frequently being more than a year old. Bayly and
Carter (2004) piloted a generic model that identified 'at-risk' female
patients aged 65+ years by questionnaire-driven case finding, and

pinpointed younger patients by the use of specific database searches. In addition to this case-finding approach, patients were offered peripheral DXA scanning where appropriate to refine their risk further. Using this approach 5% of the population (3655 from an overall population of 71 433) were identified as being at risk, of which about a quarter had BMD measurements within the osteoporotic range. After identification and appropriate intervention, the fracture rate at the initial pilot practice was followed and between years 1 and 3 there was a 55% reduction of all fractures in women aged over 65 years. It has, however, been suggested that this rate was achieved only because this specific practice had strong data quality policies, ensuring sufficient patient exposure to interventions.

In addition to the logistics of performing selective case finding in primary care, there is also the problem of accessing DXA scans to confirm the diagnosis of osteoporosis in those at risk. The NOS (2002) estimates that the number of bone density scans required, as part of a selective case-finding approach, is 1000 scans per 100 000 population. The NOS has conducted a survey to assess whether current DXA provision in the UK is sufficient to satisfy current need. Preliminary results of this survey indicate average waiting time of 18 weeks for a scan, with haphazard location of DXA machines, variation in provision of qualified staff to operate the machines and scanners being inadequately funded to operate at full clinical capacity.

In addition to selective case finding, the ideal management of osteoporosis in primary care would include preventive strategies for those at high risk, general education on bone health and initiatives to promote long-term adherence to therapy for those diagnosed with osteoporosis. The achievement of this would rest on the combined skills of GPs, all community-based nurses, physiotherapists, pharmacists and health promotion staff. Although not impossible, resource and financial implications are vast and it would also require training and education of the diverse groups involved.

The National Osteoporosis Society

The National Osteoporosis Society (NOS) is a much respected, major, national health charity, with a turnover approaching £5 million per annum and a membership of 27 000, comprising people living with

osteoporosis, their families, carers, and clinical and research professionals. The NOS employs 49 staff in two direct service delivery and
four support departments and is assisted by almost 1000 volunteers
across the UK in 130 local support groups. The charity has an enviable
clinical reputation, support and expertise and this model is mirrored
through the work of the International Osteoporosis Foundation and
sister osteoporosis organizations throughout the world. With respect
to membership services, the charity offers information via a comprehensive range of leaflets, newsletters, public meetings and a helpline,
staffed by nurse specialists. New services to be introduced over the
next 5 years include lifestyle and self-management courses and information on advocacy and patient rights. Health-care professionals can
access a full range of information leaflets, NOS position statements on
specific topics e.g. use of DXA, and a quarterly journal.

In addition the charity also provides a formal network for health professionals and organizes a prestigious conference every 18 months. The
NOS funds research projects on various aspects of osteoporosis, offers
two annual studentships and also commits to specific time-limited
projects on chosen topics. Other areas of work within NOS encompass
fundraising activities, communications with the media, contributions
to scientific topics, e.g. the National Institute for Health and Clinical
Excellence (NICE), and political lobbying to maintain and improve
services for osteoporosis. Like many other charities, the NOS is operating in uncertain and challenging times, being governed by varied
external and internal influences. Its aims for the future are to move
towards a more balanced focus and service provision to enhance its
effectiveness as a patient-centred charity. In doing so it hopes to
achieve its new vision of 'A society where prevention, treatment and
care of people with osteoporosis is of the highest standard and consistently available'.

Secondary care provision of osteoporosis services is delivered by
varied disciplines, including orthopaedics, rheumatology, care of elderly people and endocrinology. Although some services are well
established with defined referral criteria, documented protocols and
ready access to DXA, others remain fragmented and under-resourced.
Recommendations on the integration of falls and osteoporosis services
have been made in Standard 6 of the NSF for Older People, but it is
still too early to confirm whether or not this has been enacted on a

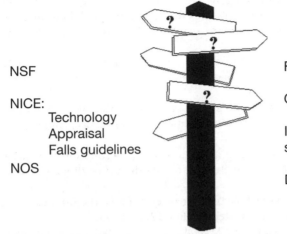

NSF

NICE:
    Technology
    Appraisal
    Falls guidelines

NOS

Fracture clinic liaison

Orthogeriatric care

Integrated falls and OP
services

DXA access

Figure 7.2 Osteoporosis services: the future. DXA, dual energy X-ray absorptiometry; NICE, National Institute for Health and Clinical Excellence; NOS, National Osteoporosis Society; NSF, National Service Framework; OP, osteoporosis.

universal basis. Within primary care the management of osteoporosis faces many competing demands and currently is not a high priority (Figure 7.2).

It is hoped that existing models of service provision will motivate, stimulate and support all health-care professionals in developing their own models that will serve to address the growing problem of osteoporosis and fractures.

The contact details for the NOS are: Camerton, Bath BA2 0PJ; tel: 01761 471771; website: www.nos.org.uk

References

Andrade SE, Majumdar SP, Chan KA et al. (2003) Low frequency of treatment among postmenopausal women following a fracture. Arch Intern Med 163: 2052–7.

Barton J, Worcester G, Ryan PJ (2003) Long term treatment adherence from a fracture liaison clinic. Osteopor Int 14(suppl 4): S12.

Bayly J, Carter G (2004) A primary care approach to managing patients at risk of osteoporotic fracture. Osteopor Rev 12(2): 7–11.

Cameron ID, Handholl HH, Finnegan TP, Madhok R, Langhorne P (2001) Coordinated multidisciplinary approaches for in patient rehabilitation of older patients with proximal femoral fracture. Cochrane Database Systematic Review (3): CD000106.

Canagon S, St Clair M, Fraser K, Wheatley T (2003) Long term management of people with fragility fracture is inadequate; an audit from mid Sussex UK. Osteopor Int 14(suppl 1): S448.

Charalambous CP, Kumar S, Tryfonides M et al. (2002) Management of osteoporosis in an orthopaedic department. Audit improves practice. Int J Clin Pract 56: 620–1.

Department of Health (1999) Making a Difference. Strengthening the nursing, midwifery and health visiting contribution to health and healthcare. London: Department of Health.

Edlington C, O'Brien K (2004) Risk factors for osteoporosis: the implications for an inner city primary care trust. Osteopor Rev 12(1): 8–11.

Gallagher AP, McQuillian CA, Harkness M, Gallacher SJ (2004) Drug compliance: inpatient hip fractures following discharge. Osteopor Int 14(suppl 4): S54.

McClellan AR, Gallacher SJ, Fraser M (2003) The fracture liaison service: success of a programme for the evaluation and management of patients with osteoporotic fracture. Osteopor Int 14:1028–34.

Marsh D, Simpson H, Wallace A (2003). The Care of Fragility Fractures. Academic Board of Orthopaedic Surgeons of the British Orthopaedic Association (BOA). London: BOA.

National Osteoporosis Society (2002) Primary Care Strategy for Osteoporosis and Falls. A framework for health improvement programmes implementing the National Service Framework for Older People. Bath: NOS.

National Osteoporosis Society (2004) All Party Parliamentary Osteoporosis Group (APPOG). Falling short: Delivering Integrated Falls and Osteoporosis Services in England. A report on the implementation of Standard Six of the National Service Framework for Older People. Bath: NOS.

National Institute for Health and Clinical Excellence (2005) Secondary Prevention of Osteoporotic Fracture in Postmenopausal Women. Guidance 87. London: NICE.

O'Neill K, Worcester G, Ryan PJ (2004) Secondary prevention following hip fracture. Osteopor Int 14(suppl 4): S58.

Shenton S, Wood A, Mackay K (2004) Do we look for osteoporosis following a low trauma fracture? Osteopor Int 14(suppl 4): S46.

Simonelli C, Chen YT, Morarley J, Lewis AF, Abbott TA (2003) Evaluation and management of osteoporosis following hospitalization for low impact fracture. J Gen Intern Med 18: 17–22.

Index